The Coping Crisis

Discover why coping skills are required for a healthy and fulfilling life

WILLIAM A. HOWATT

Foreword by Gillian Livingston from *The Globe and Mail*

ISBN 978-1-926460-03-1

Published 2015

Morneau Shepell, Ltd.
895 Don Mills Road Tower One, Suite 700
Toronto, ON M3C 1W3
www.morneaushepell.com

Cover design by Kathryn Marcellino www.custom-graphic-design.com

Dedication

I am dedicating this book to my mother, Lydia Howatt, who has always been the one person who listened to me, never judged me and helped me navigate what I suspected seemed to her like a daily coping crisis as a youth and young adult. She helped me learn to believe in myself and to learn we can only create what we believe is possible. As a result, I have learned how to cope with the demands of life — well, most days — as there is no such thing as perfect. Nevertheless, she has been a force to remind me that I can make my thinking become my reality.

Thanks, Mom.

Love, Bill

Additional praise for *The Coping Crisis*

Despite being an affluent society, general unhappiness and feelings of low self-esteem have never been more prevalent. In both patients and healthcare workers, the inability to cope with life's daily challenges is a major cause of these negative feelings. As with any illness, it is essential to understand the problem and to become accountable. Bill Howatt's book takes us into the life of a typical person who is unable to cope with life's daily challenges. By linking coping ability to mental wellness, and by defining and slowing "coping churn," the author has provided me with some tools that will be useful in helping my patients to address their behaviour and its effect on their disease states. It is now much clearer to me that most of my patients and unhealthy co-workers have an inability to cope — something I had never been able to clearly explain, until I read this book.

~Marc Pelletier, MD, MSc, FRCSC. Head, Division of Cardiac Surgery, New Brunswick Heart Centre

Stress is something we all experience on a daily basis. Dr. Howatt's book *The Coping Crisis* helps us not only better understand stress but, more importantly, how to effectively deal and cope with the inevitable stressors we encounter on a daily basis. It is the book I recommend to anyone looking for a practical roadmap to becoming a better self-coach and who wants to continue to develop personally and/or professionally.

~Dave Veale, Founder and CEO, Vision Coaching Inc.

Dr. Bill Howatt has opened my eyes to the staggering societal impacts associated with workplace stress. His latest book, *The Coping Crisis*, walks you through the causes, symptoms and impacts associated with mental health issues in the workplace, but more importantly provides mechanisms to both identify workplace stressors and introduce new coping skills. Bill has brought a new level of passion, science and rigour to the field of work-life impacts and the need to create new coping pathways for individuals and employees.

~Neil Jacobsen, Commissioner, Strategic Services, City of Saint John

The viewpoint of life through Sam's eyes provides the reader with a simplistic understanding of how difficult life is when one has gaps in their coping skills. We come to know Sam through his personal journey and are able to better understand how many of those around us may be going through the same or similar crisis. Dr. Howatt's straightforward approach, combined with language that is easily understood, is refreshing, yet informative and educational. I would personally recommend that anyone struggling to cope, or anyone who knows of someone who may be, should read this book to gain a better understanding of the indicators and the strategies available.

~Ian D. Allen, Executive Director, College of Extended Learning,
University of New Brunswick

As a CEO leading a company that ultimately empowers people to take a proactive and engaged approach to wellness living, I fully appreciate the significant challenges in front of anyone who is trying to change their self-destructive behaviours. Bill Howatt's book has enlightened me on the significance of arming people with appropriate coping skills that will see them through challenging moments and ultimately lead people to choose a path of "change" rather than "convenience." This is a book that should be shared with everybody — across any age, demographic or population. Whether you are a type 2 diabetic or an aspiring Olympian, Bill's strategies and mechanisms can be leveraged to achieve true change and long-lasting results.

I would highly recommend this book for anybody who is looking to make meaningful change in their life and develop the appropriate mental tools to cope with any situation presented to them.

~Dr. Travis McDonough, Founder and CEO, Kinduct Technologies

Bill Howatt proves once again that knowledge is power, with a peek behind the curtain of human behaviour to explore how our beliefs construct our lives. He then shows us a way forward to systematically unleash our potential. An insightful and practical read for individuals, teams and organizations.

~Janice MacInnis, Manager, Organizational Health, Dalhousie University

Thanks to the great work of many Canadians who are passionate about raising awareness of mental health issues, like the Canadian Mental Health Association and the Mental Health Commission of Canada, many people are much more open about discussing mental health and mental illness, and there are many national campaigns on this theme. However, talking about mental illness doesn't seem to be making Canadians healthier. In fact, statistics on the prevalence of mental illnesses and the impact in workplaces suggest that it is a growing problem — and yet, there is more being done to support mental health than ever before. These trends have been the focus of many studies, including one conducted by a partnership between *The Globe and Mail* and Dr. Bill Howatt. The data suggests that rather than seeing these trends as pointing to a mental health crisis, we need to recognize that this is a coping crisis. Just as a public campaign for public hygiene can greatly reduce the development of epidemics, a campaign for mental health hygiene in the form of promoting healthy coping skills can greatly reduce an epidemic of depression and anxiety in the population. By sharing Sam's journey, as told in this book, we can better understand the relationship between coping skills and mental health.

~C. Robinson, HR Manager in a Canadian Acute Care Health Facility

★★★

Wonderful book — very relevant and helpful to employers, employees, individuals, parents and students.

~Reid Estey Head of HR, Saint Francis Xavier University

★★★

As a labour and employment lawyer, I've dealt with countless workplace disputes that are fuelled by stress. Managers under pressure to meet benchmarks behave abrasively and then abusively toward employees; employees whose nerves are frayed by personal issues such as debt or marital breakdowns become poor performers at work; both managers and employees who feel threatened in their positions engage in organizationally disruptive behaviour as a means of self-protection; and the list goes on. Bill Howatt has extensively studied workplace stress issues and, in this book, offers insights that will help anyone who is weighed down with stress to cope. *The Coping Crisis* is an important gateway to a more tranquil existence.

~Kelly VanBuskirk, Ph.D., C.Arb. (P.C.) Lawson Creamer

Table of Contents

Acknowledgements

I would like to make a special mention for Al Kingsbury, who played a critical role in assisting me to take my words and shape them for this book. Without Al's support and patience this book would not have happened. Why? I have lived my entire life with dyslexia and ADHD and I understand the pain of failure, how difficult life can be, and the benefits of coping skills. There may be no one activity more difficult in the world for me than writing. It was not until I developed a set of strategies and have become comfortable and confident to ask for help to transform my ideas onto paper in a format that others can read that I was able to begin writing books. Thanks, Al, for getting me through more than one of these projects.

I would also like to acknowledge and thank all the reviewers who took time out of their busy schedules to share their thoughts, comments and edits. Thank you for your praise and support for *The Coping Crisis* as an important topic to explore. Finally, I would like to give a special thank you to Gillian Livingston for her contribution to this book and support in helping me help employees better cope with stress through the Your Life at Work Study through *The Globe and Mail*, and Greg Caines for his passion and commitment to talk to employers and employees about what they can do to curb the coping crisis.

Foreword

"So, how are you doing?"

Nowadays, there are so many layers behind this simple question asked around the water cooler at work. It asks, "How are you coping?"; "How are you managing?"; "How's your workload?"; "Is your manager being fair?"; "How's your work-life balance?"

Anyone who works knows that life has changed, usually not for the better, in the past decade or more at the typical workplace in Canada. We are asked to do more with less, faster, with more consequences for errors. Many organizations are trying to run as tight a ship as possible. There are no "excess" workers. Everyone's workload is much heavier than before. We've been through recessions and layoffs and have felt the repercussions when staff members are let go and their workload has simply been spread amongst those who remain.

As a result, workers are stressed. Their managers are stressed and put more pressure on those working for them. Employees are trying to meet tougher deadlines at work while trying to balance those demands with the needs of their spouses and families. It puts workers in a bind and without effective coping skills, it can send some people over the edge — first from not being able to manage their life and work, to feeling stressed, to frustrated and then stressed to the max. When that happens, no one benefits and the employee suffers the most.

Seeing this change in people's working lives was the basis for *The Globe and Mail's* Your Life at Work survey, done in conjunction with Bill Howatt. Bill and I took his 300+ Quality of Work Life questionnaire and whittled it down to a mini version. We then watched as more than 7,000 people took our online survey from February 2014 to January 2015. It was clear from the response from readers that stress and finding ways to manage work and life stressors were issues that hit a chord with working Canadians. Follow the link for a detailed summary of the findings: www.theglobeandmail.com/report-on-business/careers/career-advice/life-at-work/survey-says-were-stressed-and-not-loving-it/article22722102/.

The survey of more than 7,300 Canadians found that 60 percent of workers felt stressed and were struggling to cope with the demands of their work and private lives. The demands and atmosphere at work were found to be key drivers of stress, such as job expectations, a lack of trust between management and staff, gossiping, peer interaction and culture.

Those who felt the most stressed indicated that they did not have strong coping skills and put in less effort on a day-to-day basis, called in sick more often and were less engaged at work. Stressed employees were also more likely to turn to harmful ways of managing their stress, such as overeating, drinking alcohol, gambling or using illegal drugs.

However, on the flip side, those who felt their stress was under control showed they had better coping skills, were more engaged with their work, were happier, more fulfilled, more productive and healthier. The survey also found that the cost to businesses if they ignored the health and well-being of their staff could be in the millions of dollars due to increased sick days, higher benefit costs and loss of productivity.

When you put it all together, the survey showed that organizations can benefit from better supporting their employees and helping staff improve their coping skills to ensure that workplaces keep the health and welfare of their staff top of mind.

The fact is few people do any formal training to improve their coping skills, which includes learning to manage emotions, deal with stressors, handle pressure and expectations and manage time. These skills are gradually learned throughout the school and work years, or you may struggle later on. And it's often a sink-or-swim proposition. If you can balance your time and manage expectations, you'll get a decent mark on your school project or satisfy your boss at work. But if you're not taught how to do that, and just thrown a task in the hopes you'll figure it out, there may be some challenges.

In addition to hiring effective managers and keeping work-loads reasonable, if workplaces can help their staff learn better coping skills, such as how to effectively deal with managers, manage their time, balance home and work responsibilities, relieve stress through exercise and other activities — they can help their staff be more productive, happier and less stressed people.

Anyone who has ever been in a managerial position for any time knows how stress affects staff. From the one worker who can handle only one task at a time and needs every request spelled out in detail, to the staffer you know can handle a workload three times that of his colleague, you know how coping skills are key to workplace productivity. A workplace needs to be fair, for certain, but you can also help staff cope with the stresses of life and work that the workplace can't always control.

Workplaces everywhere in this day and age can be challenging, and the more we can create effective workplaces and help workers cope with the demands placed upon them by work and private life, the better we all will be.

This book's focus is on behavioural-based coping skills. These are skills that can be taught to help a person cope better with stress. They impact how effectively one can problem solve, make decisions, deal with pressure, control emotions, push through adversity to achieve a goal, deal with conflict, recover from failure, adapt to change, move past rejections, manage workloads and believe in their ability to control their own destiny. These are all outcomes of a person who has well-developed coping skills.

How one copes with life ultimately defines one's success. This book breaks down the coping crisis with respect to how it happens and what a person like Sam can do to cope with various scenarios. Sam is the fictional character that is described throughout the book to help the reader explore the concepts of coping. Each chapter provides ideas for people like Sam or those who are interested in assisting people like him.

That's why this book is important right now — the working world is at a crossroads. Organizations need employees to be productive, but they're forgetting that people are not machines and have more to their lives than just work. Businesses must see the economic sense it makes to treat their employees well, keep workloads reasonable, hire effective managers, offer generous vacations and commit to having an open and honest workplace culture. And workers need to know how vital it is to their own health and well-being to be able to manage the stress that comes with work and life. Employees must know that they need to speak up to be able to better manage the demands on them, and they need to find a balance of some sort between work and life. The productivity of organizations around the world and employees is at stake.

~Gillian Livingston, former Careers Editor,
Assistant Editor, Globe Investor, The Globe and Mail

Preface

I have been working in the health and benefits industry for the past 23 years and have seen lots of change and trends during that time. In the 90s, employers witnessed annual double-digit cost pressures as new, revolutionary drugs came to market. Many drugs emerged in completely new categories matched to new lifestyle related ailments (I have spoken to many physicians over the years who continue to assert that 75 percent of the health issues they see in their offices every day are due to lifestyle choices). There are drugs to control heartburn when we overeat or drink too much coffee. High cholesterol counts resulting from poor food habits are treated with new drugs. When we feel a bit blue, we can get an antidepressant…wait a minute…this last one feels a bit different than the first two, but we'll come back to that in a second.

During the 2000s we saw a variety of cost-containment strategies to tackle the cost pressures from the prior decade. As the 2000s were coming to a close we began to see the arrival of specialty and biologic medications. These biologics have transformed patient care for many severe and debilitating conditions. They also represent a significant new cost for employers and plan sponsors (incidentally, while saving provincial hospital budgets vast sums of money due to reductions in surgeries and quietly deflecting care from in-patient/outpatient to in-home). Generic drug price reforms and multiple brand medication patent expiries marked the early 2010s and provided welcome cost relief for many plan sponsors. Reforms on generics pricing may have temporarily masked the emerging cost concerns represented by the specialty and biologic drug class that will continue to be a major cost driver in the future.

Why am I telling you this? Well, employers have played an important role in the health and wellbeing of employees' lives for as long as I can remember through their involvement in employee benefits. In addition to benefits programs, many employers also offer a wide array of programs and initiatives under what they may call the "employee wellness" umbrella. Unfortunately, in most cases the business impact of these wellness initiatives is not measured, leaving decision-makers and finance to wonder about ROI or outcome measurement. In many cases, employers feel they are preaching to the converted as the 10 percent of employees that choose to participate are already involved in pro-health activities.

I presented at a human resources conference earlier this year with a well-known workplace health consultant who also happens to be a physician. He essentially pleaded with the audience of HR professionals to stop their "random acts of wellness." His comments received a few embarrassed chuckles but the kernel of truth in his plea leads me to my next question, "What IS the employer's role as it relates to employee health and wellness?"

Here's a possible answer. Employers cannot *fix* employees but rather, they can facilitate an opportunity for employees to help themselves (e.g., promote and facilitate psychological safe workplaces). For an employee to take charge of their health and fulfillment each employee will first need to take accountability for their own health. For many organizations, creating a shared accountability model with their employees is the desired cultural direction for the future. It recognizes that there are things the employer can do to foster a physically and mentally healthy work environment and it recognizes there are things employees need to own and be accountable for related to their health and productivity. A tall order for certain, given the expectations and entitlements we have fostered over the past decades. "There's a pill for whatever ails us" needs to evolve or the current model will not be sustainable. I'm not suggesting medications don't play an important part in our healthcare system, they do, what I'm suggesting is that we as individuals will be healthier when we first learn to care for our minds and bodies in order that we have the capacity and energy to be the best version of ourselves for the benefit of our families, communities and workplaces.

Back to my story about antidepressants. The worldwide success of these drugs underscored the significance and growth of mental health issues in mainstream society and at least started to get the conversation out of the closet. Since that time, many medications used to treat depression, anxiety and bipolar disorder, to name a few, have come into widespread use. The evidence is clear. For the majority of employers, mental health medications are often the number one or number two most used drug class by number of prescriptions in their covered populations. Often, the most common cause of employee absence both short term and long term is due to mental health challenges. In the workplace, aggressive behaviour and bullying are on the rise and employee engagement scores continue to perplex many organizational leaders.

I was speaking at a Conference Board of Canada event recently to a group of large national employers. I asked them by show of hands who was measuring employee engagement. The majority of hands shot up. I then asked how many of them had as an organizational imperative to improve employee engagement scores. Again, most hands were raised. I then asked the group, "Is it possible we're measuring the wrong thing?" The reaction to which was a buzz of chatter and piqued curiosity. A bit facetious, perhaps, but the point I was trying to make is that something else comes before engagement and that's our ability to think, problem solve and process the many stressors, both real and perceived, that come at us every minute of every day. When we hire employees, we typically seek candidates who have the right mix of education, work experience and personal attributes but we often do not assess their ability to think and reason, especially under stressful circumstances. In many situations, we don't often appreciate a person's ability to cope under stress until long after they are on the job.

Thanks to organizations like Bell Canada, who are demonstrating through leadership how to talk about mental health in the workplace, the conversation is evolving into action. And while emphasis has tended to be placed on the most serious organic mental health issues faced by one in five Canadians, the truth of the matter is that we are all somewhere on the mental wellness continuum as illustrated below with the majority of us on any given day in the frustrated category or worse. And if you are familiar with the stress-strain relationship you will know that a mind under stress for extended periods of time will result in the body breaking down. Not the outcome anyone wants but unless we understand what we can do to prevent this downward slide this is our probable fate.

The premise on which this book is based is that we don't have a mental health crisis in Canada; we have a "coping skills crisis." It's the classic "chicken or egg story." I know what you're probably thinking, enough of "the sky is falling" talk already! Well, I am very optimistic about the resilience of human beings and our innate ability to rise to the occasion. Employers have an opportunity to play an important role in reshaping the future trajectory of employee health that reaches beyond the workplace and into our communities by not trying to "fix" employees but by facilitating an opportunity for employees to help themselves. A two-way conversation that results in employers being better at what they can influence such as leadership training/development and clear policies administered consistently such as antibullying and harassment while employees are accountable for their end of the conversation in managing their health and productivity. And so as you read this book and the story of Sam I would ask you think about what Sam and his employer could do differently to drive a better outcome.

~Greg Caines, Partner, Morneau Shepell

CHAPTER 1

The Challenge

Honk…honk honk…honk honk honk honk honk!!!

It's 7:00 p.m. Sam sits quietly at a three-light intersection, gazing through his windshield at the setting sun reflecting off the water on a perfectly clear evening. On the surface, it appears that he's taking in the perfect backdrop on his way home from another day of work; however, on the inside Sam's mind is critiquing his day. He says to himself, "It's happening again. My mind is running all over the place about work. Why doesn't it stop?"

The light turns green but Sam doesn't shift his gaze as he waits for an internal response to his question. After several seconds, the driver of a large red 4x4 truck directly behind Sam is keen to get rolling. He hits his horn with a respectful single and two honks combination — as polite as a honk can be. The driver's first intentions are simple: a gesture to encourage Sam's little white car to move on. Sam doesn't react, he just keeps gazing. His mind is distracted as he processes the events of the day.

The truck driver moves from polite honks to a steady blaring of his horn. This startles Sam and brings him back from his mental journey; his mind moves from being in park to forward gear. A feeling of embarrassment comes over him and with it a rush of adrenalin. As well, from somewhere deep in his mind comes an option for action. *I should tell this person off so they leave me alone."*

But Sam quickly re-thinks, *"If I say that, he may want to fight and I don't want to fight, I just want to get out of this situation now."* With that, Sam's thoughts of being aggressive fade. He's frustrated, shaken and upset, but he has a long history of being able to bottle up his emotions to reduce his risk for conflict.

"OK, I don't want any conflict here. I just need to get moving and get this person off my back," Sam thinks, as he turns his focus to the task at hand. He sits up in his seat, shakes his head, looks around to ensure the intersection is clear, and slowly moves forward. He's starting to gain his composure and his rush is subsiding.

As Sam proceeds, he notices the driver behind shaking his head, showing his disapproval. Sam doesn't react to the driver's nonverbal gestures. He's preoccupied with getting his mind back on driving and processing what just happened. As he moves up the street a few blocks, he thinks to himself, *"It happened again. My mind is running all over the place about work. Why do I keep letting this job get to me? For heaven's sake, I can't even drive a car without feeling stressed."*

Sam had another tough day at work, which happens to be his "normal." He was working all day on Project Thales, the code name for his current IT project. This project has been complex and ended up being much more work than was originally anticipated. Sam has been working on it for several weeks, with the timeline for the final deliverable in four days. But today his manager moved the timeline up without any notice.

His manager called him into his office at 4:00 p.m. to tell Sam that the client wanted the timeline moved up two days, which he agreed to without consulting Sam. This was a shock to Sam. Four days was going to be a push; two days would require a massive effort. What made things even more complex for Sam was that he couldn't do anything more to advance the project at this time. He was waiting for more materials that would not get to him until the next morning. Now he had to figure out how to get four days of complex work done in two days. The stakes and pressure had been amped up and he was exasperated as he walked out of the office. Nevertheless, as frustrated as he was he didn't let his manager know he was upset. He took the news quietly and walked out of the office.

Work has been difficult for Sam over the past several years. He typically feels under pressure due to what he believes are excessive work demands and a controlling manager. His job is packed with looming deadlines and high expectations that he will deliver results. He perceives that he is never asked his opinion, just told what to do and by when. He feels that the daily norm is for him to pull the proverbial rabbit out of a hat and make what seems the impossible happen — without any regard to the hardships brought upon him. The pressure of the job keeps his mind running on lists of things to do that are top of mind for him most every waking moment. Unless he's watching TV, his mind feels as if it's focused on work 24-7.

Sam often leaves these conversations with his boss feeling as though his manager is talking down to him and showing him no respect. He knows that he's the only person on the information technology team that can pull all the pieces together to close out these kinds of complex, multistep projects. However, he has yet to find a way to express his concerns to his manager; he simply keeps things bottled up inside. He often asks himself how he's going to keep up the torrid work pace, because he's finding work demands exhausting. It's common for him to be in the office by 7:30 a.m. and working until 7:00 p.m. The long hours and high work demands are taking a toll on him.

Once Sam pulls into his driveway he pauses and says to himself, "I find it frustrating. It's a perfect evening and I can't seem to see any joy in it and I don't have a clue how to relax." At this point he would simply convince himself that life is unfair and difficult. Onlookers would describe Sam as reserved, certainly not an outgoing and happy person.

On a daily basis, Sam spends an inordinate amount of mental energy thinking about how hard he is finding his work and his lack of job fulfillment in his current role. He feels torn. He loves IT, but he doesn't like how he's being managed. He would like to see some recognition from his manager or, at the very least, hear his manager ask him what he thinks and feel confident that if he questioned his manager he would be treated respectfully.

As Sam heads for work each day it's not uncommon for him to wonder how he will be able to get through the day. "This job is too hard," he thinks. Perhaps the one thing that keeps him coming back is he likes IT and knows he's good at it. These internal conversations are the source of much of his tension and stress. But not all; there's another source of stress that also eats at Sam.

Sam is a quiet and kind person who lives alone. His life is simple: he has work and work alone. No pets, partner or close friends. He waves at his neighbours each morning when their paths cross but he rarely talks to any of them other than simple salutations and general comments about the weather and current news. He doesn't even know the names of most his neighbours; he just recognizes them.

For most of his life, Sam has done as much as he can to avoid conflict. As a result, he hasn't taken many chances. The past 10 years have flown by. He has a history of chronic stress and today he's struggling with several health issues. Between the ages of 34 and 39 he put an extra 60 pounds on his 5'10" body due to a poor diet and night snacking supported by a sedentary lifestyle that involved no physical activity. He now weighs 230 pounds. At age 39 he was put on hypertension medication, and two years later he was diagnosed as being clinically depressed. Now 42, he was recently diagnosed as a type 1 diabetic (late onset), so he now has several chronic diseases, most of which likely could have been prevented.

Sam continues to live the same lifestyle. His doctor has discussed his concerns with regard to Sam's health and life choices on numerous occasions. While health and happiness sound like compelling concepts, they are not in Sam's line of sight as ever being possible. Happiness in Sam's mind is something other people have found. He missed his chance. He perceives his current health issues as mostly due to bad luck. He has failed to accept or perhaps fully understand how his lifestyle choices have played a major role in defining and creating his current state of health. He has not yet processed how coping skills or the lack thereof played a role in the choices he has made thus far in this life.

Today, this 42-year-old is starting to ask himself more existential questions with regard to the meaning of life. His reality on a typical day involves spending many more hours alone than with people. When alone he feels he has been dealt a poor hand in life. He doesn't see anything changing for him and he often feels powerless to make any real change. He often runs the internal script that it's too late to change his life. His course has been set; he sees no positives in his future. Unknowingly, he's trapped in a self-fulfilling prophecy.

Sam grew up in a family where both parents worked and he was an only child. His parents were kind to Sam, but didn't have much time for him. He also doesn't recall much, if any, affection or acknowledgement. As a result, he has few positive family memories. Sam learned as a child not to be a distraction to his parents; they appeared to Sam to be happiest when they didn't hear from him. Sam's childhood memories are quite tragic since he believes as a child he was never treated with love nor celebrated on any level. Nor does he have any happy memories.

Sam has no surviving family members today. Both of his parents have passed; he feels alone in the world with no family support system.

As a youth, Sam always struggled socially to cope with peer pressure. He was bullied, which resulted in learning to avoid conflict and people. He never had an opportunity nor was in a position to develop assertiveness or conflict management skills. From an early age he has felt that the environment defines and controls his fate. One of the best ways for him to get along in life is to not draw attention to himself, but rather to do his work and keep to himself.

At work he's known as the odd, fat, quiet IT guy. No one bugs Sam. But no one is really close to him, either. A few of his colleagues speak IT with him, but that's the extent of his social interactions. His weight used to bother him but he has accepted that he's obese and always will be.

When confronted with a life challenge, it's typical for Sam to become overwhelmed on the inside but show no emotion on the outside. He has mastered the art of showing no emotion when upset. He keeps his emotions inside and looks for an escape plan from what he perceives to be the cause of his stress. Once he feels his internal panic button turn on he does all he can to reduce his risk of facing further stress or conflict by escaping. His strategy is simple: avoid and run. As a teen, Sam found conflict or the threat of conflict with peers stressful. As a result, he didn't participate in

Being in control of your life and having realistic expectations about your day-to-day challenges are the keys to stress management, which is perhaps the most important ingredient to living a happy, healthy and rewarding life. — Marilu Henner

team sports, date or engage in social activities. He threw himself into his school work, putting in hour upon hour doing homework. He became a top student, graduating from high school with a 93 percent grade point average.

Being a straight "A" student in high school, Sam carried this on to undergraduate school where he received a B.Sc. in engineering and a Masters in Computer Engineering. His teachers always enjoyed Sam. He was the perfect student: on time, did his work and was not demanding. Sam never complained and seldom asked for anything. He excelled in his education; it was his number one focus. Sam also knew he was good at school. It was the fuel that kept him going.

Over the years, Sam ended up on a few dates in his twenties and early thirties that were the result of one lovely young woman asking him out. Recently, however, that has not happened. It's been seven years since he was on a date. To this day, Sam finds dealing with, or even the thought of dealing with, another person's expectations and demands overwhelming. He wishes it could be different but has accepted that being alone is easier, less complex and less stressful. He definitely fits the profile of an introvert and loner. He has also given up on the notion that anyone would want to be with him or love him as he is.

Sam started this job basically right out of graduate school at age 26, although he had a few part-time roles before this full-time position. Even after years of creating a positive track record in the IT field he still lacks the confidence to push back on his manager or believe he could do better in his career. As a result, he feels trapped in his job. He doesn't think anyone would hire him and he thinks it's best to not push his luck. For the past 16 years, to the best of his recollection, he has felt miserable 90 percent of the time.

Sam has learned that it's paramount for him to take the path with the least amount of risk. He continues to avoid people and places. Within two years of starting his job Sam began to feel trapped. At 42 he still feels trapped.

To escape from the pain of feeling trapped in a job where he felt powerless, Sam began to use food as a way to cope with work stress. He engaged in the unhealthy behaviour of eating at night for emotional symptom relief. This was the start of his coping crisis.

> We acquire the strength we have overcome. When it is dark enough, you can see the stars. All life is an experiment. The more experiments you make the better. — Ralph Waldo Emerson

A coping crisis occurs when a person's internal resources are not sufficient to support them in managing the demands being put on them by life or themselves. The longer a person stays in a coping crisis, the higher their risk for developing a chronic disease such as mental illness.

For most of his life, Sam has felt he has been under chronic stress and has been powerless to get what he really wants. He would like to be in a loving relationship, have friends and enjoy the people around him, but how to do this and cope with all his perceived life challenges has been and continues to be a barrier.

Sam's manager may not tell him to his face but his employer values Sam's talent and work ethic. They know Sam is their ace for solving complex IT engineering problems. The manager's character flaws are evident when he shares his belief that Sam has a low confidence level and that Sam's happiness is not his concern; he's Sam's manager, not his therapist. The manager shows little to no empathy for Sam. An onlooker may suggest this manager treats Sam like a machine more than a person with feelings and needs.

The manager knows Sam does the work of three people most days. He's OK to see Sam put forth a high discretionary effort each and every day with no sense of need to acknowledge him, and he has shown little to no interest in Sam's health. When Sam calls in sick or goes to one of his numerous medical appointments the manager never questions him. He acts as if it's understood that Sam will be back and will make up the lost time.

To Sam's credit, he never complains about his manager. He's a private person who keeps his personal matters inside. He never complains to anyone but himself about his life, and he's never pushed back on his manager's demands. He works as hard as he can each and every day. The only signal that something may be wrong is his declining health. His employer doesn't know what Sam is thinking or feeling, most likely because no one has asked, and his manager has made no attempt to engage Sam on a personal level; he takes him for granted. Sam and his manager have worked together from the start. Sam has endured 16 years of coming to work every day dealing with a manager who doesn't inspire him and whom he really doesn't trust.

The manager knows Sam is struggling with a few health issues, based on his time off for medical appointments. He also knows that Sam gets along with his peers on the surface but he hasn't developed any strong relationships; he's viewed as a loner. Sam's approach to life is to be quiet, agreeable and follow instructions well. He doesn't show any emotion. For example, his manager has no clue that Sam doesn't respect, trust or like him. Sam's peers seem to be fine with him and treat him with respect; they all know he's an IT thought leader and a real problem solver. Nonetheless, no one has gotten close to Sam. He's viewed as a nice guy who is a recluse who wants to be left alone. Most of his peers would know he's a diabetic because they observe him testing his blood and taking insulin at work.

What Sam's manager and peers are unaware of is the number of hours Sam spends dealing with his regret and thinking about his work: how alone he feels and how much his current station in life is eating at him. There's a good chance some of his peers would have lots of empathy for Sam if they knew he wanted more social interaction. Sam is silently experiencing a coping crisis.

Sadly, Sam is not atypical. Many adults struggle to find peace and happiness and to escape loneliness. The root cause of Sam's life challenges at work and at home is a gap in his ability to cope. He's experiencing a coping crisis.

The next chapter introduces coping skills.

CHAPTER 2

Coping Skills

So what are coping skills? Coping skills support the body similar to physical fitness. For example, a person's physical fitness can be measured by strength, endurance and speed. A person's fitness level defines how well they can perform a physical task on demand. Individuals who specialize and train to run the 100-metre sprint at a competitive level train for years to run a 10-second or better race. They understand their success requires on-demand performance, meaning they turn on a switch, react and perform once the starting gun goes off. The noise of the gun is the trigger for the sprinter to fully engage their body to perform to its full potential. Many variables define a sprinter's success, such as conditioning, genetics and training.

Coping skills are similar; they are on demand, with the environment often acting as the starting gun. Consider when Sam was at the traffic light with the horn honking behind him — the starting gun. The gap between the sound of the horn and the decision not to tell off the truck driver but to safely move his car is where coping skills play an important role. Coping skills influenced what Sam did at the time, as well as what he did after. As we will learn, with Sam it's not what he does in the moment that's causing him the most risk; it's what he does later to cope with the burden and stress he perceives he's living under.

Coping skills are in essence the tools a person has to manage how they interact with their world. Like the sprinter, the better they train and practice, the greater their chances they will perform to their full potential.

How a person copes can be influenced by personality, which influences how one perceives and filters the world. Introverts and extroverts typically have a preference as to how they like to charge their batteries with respect to people. This preference may influence how they behave. It's not uncommon for an introvert to want to get away from people to have alone time, where an extrovert will seek out others to recharge their batteries. This is but one example of how personality can influence how a person copes and interacts with their environment. The challenge is that it's difficult to change personality. Attempting to change one's personality is often ineffective. They can be aware of their

"Over and over, the data shows us that it is the Sams that have the highest employee benefit costs. It is not surprising that organizations investing in wellness programs want to reach the Sams within their population. But despite the incentives to participate, the creative health initiatives and the education offered, these employers are frustrated as rarely can the Sams be enticed to participate. Perhaps wellness programs have not been focusing on the right intervention for the people in Sam's situation? Unless Sam's coping crisis is addressed, he may not have the initiative or the ability to change lifestyle behaviours that will improve his health."

~Rochelle Morandini, B.Comm, MBA, Partner, Co-Lead of National Health Consulting, Morneau Shepell

personality and take action to modify their behaviour. The introvert can push themselves to be with people longer than they may prefer if their work requires it.

Coping Skills are Trainable

When Sam is faced with what he perceives as a life challenge (e.g., thinking about having a conversation with his manager in the coming day), he automatically moves to what's called secondary appraisal.[1] In secondary appraisal, Sam starts to pool psychological, social, time and physical resources at his disposal to cope with a situation. Once this appraisal of inventory is completed, he's left to make a choice and determine what actions he will or will not take to address his presenting external stressor.

Many people with underdeveloped coping skills become controlled by their environment. An environmental stimulus such as the honking of a horn becomes the perception as to why a person acts the way they do. For example, Jack is more aggressive than Sam. If Jack were in the same traffic situation as Sam, with a honking horn upsetting him, he likely would go from calm to a fit of rage in seconds. He would also blame the other driver for making him lose his temper.

Modern-day psychology and neuroscience are teaching that human beings can be influenced but they can't be controlled. How a person manages their life stressors is critical in predicting their future health.

People in a coping crisis may not be exactly like Sam but certainly many share unhealthy coping habits. Those who never developed coping skills are left to their own devices to find a way to cope with the life challenges they face. Coping skills are the internal intrapersonal skills one draws upon to manage themselves when faced with challenges from their environment. Coping skills are trainable; a person can be taught to cope effectively with their life challenges.

Individuals who struggle with coping often look for escapes. Sam embraces social isolation, night snacking, TV, the Internet and sleep. Perhaps without defining it, these behaviours are his best attempts to move away from stress, feel better and feel safe.

Being a bright person, Sam knows that being alone is a part of his problem. He has evolved to the point where his current life challenges and coping mechanisms have become habits and he goes into this protection mode automatically. His internal dialogue is helpless. He sadly believes he's trapped and that his life course and destiny have been set.

What we think and believe becomes our reality. Sam is creating his reality each day through his beliefs, thinking and actions. Nevertheless, he's unaware that the story he's running is what his mind believes to be true. That's one of the powerful misunderstandings for many people like Sam. They're not aware that they are writing their own story; they think outside factors are the author. But the reality is they have the pen. Sam has never learned how to effectively cope with conflict and stress on a personal and professional level.

> Do you know anyone like Sam?
>
> On the surface, does the idea Sam is experiencing a coping crisis make sense to you?

How well a person learns to cope is not based simply on genetics or personality. Coping skills are influenced by opportunities and experiences where a person learns how to deal with and manage a situation. Coping is like any skill. It's dependent on what a person has learned, mastered and practised. There are exceptions to this. For people with mental health issues such as bipolar disorder, their genetic makeup plays a major role in how well they can interact, process and cope with their environment. In Sam's case, there are no genetic issues; his issues are rooted in psychosocial choices.

The challenge for people like Sam is to become aware, consider and accept that their actions are setting their life course and if they don't learn to manage their lives more effectively, the ending will be as they wrote it. For countless people this is not a happy ending.

Coping Skills Gap

Coping skills are not simply based on common sense. Like any other skill, they need to be learned and continually practised. A large number of adults have gaps in coping skills because they basically did not formally or informally have an opportunity to focus on and practise developing their coping skills. There may not be a more important life skill for human beings than coping skills. For sure, it's right up there with math and English; it doesn't, however, get the same attention and priority in the education system.

Individuals who change their lives through cognitive behavioural therapy or self-help groups like Alcoholics Anonymous do so because they focus on developing their coping skills to better manage their lives. For many this experience changes their life. Why? They learn a new set of skills that they can apply to their lives so that all the bad stressors, triggers and events no longer upset them in the same way. They have learned the skills needed to live a healthy life. Imagine how many of these people could have avoided many life hardships if they had developed those skills before their lives became metaphorically a car wreck.

Without proper learning, guidance and practice there will be no coping mastery. The chances of being in a coping crisis like Sam's are high. In most industries, the 10-year rule is commonly accepted. This states that it typically takes a person 10 years to master a skill. It won't always take 10 years for someone with motivation to be proficient at coping; nonetheless, it does take commitment.

Like any skill, the more practice and experience, the higher the likelihood of proficiency. Coping skills support us to dampen and control powerful emotions that are created when we are fearful, stressed or overwhelmed. Figure 2-1 provides a visual overview of a theoretical model I used to frame my Quality of Work Life research.[2] The thesis of this model is people with better coping skills are less likely to experience health issues. As well, these same people will be more engaged in the workplace. This model explains why Jack and Jill — neither of whom has a genetic mental health issue — can go to the same workplace, have the same manager, shift and training, but over the years start to pick different ways to cope with work. Jack goes home and engages in unhealthy behaviours to cope, while Jill engages her

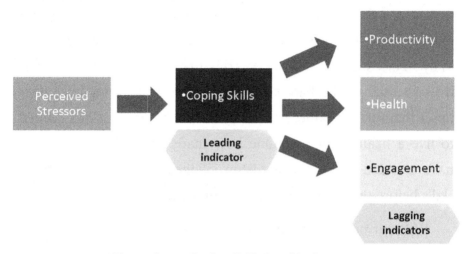

Figure 2-1 — Coping Skills Lead Indicator

family and pro-health activities like exercise and her passion for music where she sings in the local choir and coaches her daughter's hockey team. The difference between the two is their coping skills.

Every employee is challenged by workplace stressors. How they cope predicts their engagement, health and productivity. It's worth noting that employees like Sam who on the surface may appear to be highly engaged in their work are quite literally dying on the inside.

Our research through *The Globe and Mail*'s Your Life at Work[3] study found that coping skills are a leading indicator for predicting employees' level of workplace engagement and health. The higher employees' coping skills, the more likely they are content with their station in life.

What this study confirmed is the importance of coping skills for reducing one's risk for chronic disease, including mental illnesses. With the outcome from this research we started questioning whether we are asking the right questions around the growth in mental health issues.

Are we having a mental health crisis or a coping crisis? My research and professional experience have led me to the point that I think we are having a coping crisis, that a core driver for the increase in mental illness is a lack of coping skills. When a person has gaps in their coping skills and they are ineffective at dealing with their life stressors, their overall health is at risk.

The motivation for this book came out of nearly 30 years of clinical work. I believe there are many people like Sam who are caught in a coping crisis — often without knowing it until the symptoms of stress become apparent. I have determined through my work that lives can be enhanced through developing coping skills. Importantly, people need to be open and willing to make the effort. Moving past guilt associated with poor coping skills often is a step required to help a

One interesting question I have asked when talking to management and employees is, "Do we have a mental health crisis or a coping crisis?" What do you think?

person move forward. One strategy that seems to help many is to normalize that their choices are not atypical and they are not alone. It doesn't excuse the choice; it's just a fact. Many people have made poor choices trying to cope with life. If they get this point it creates an opportunity for a new conversation.

Once a person can start this new line of thinking they are open to learning and exploring what they can do better to cope with their current life challenges.

With the help of Sam's story, you have an opportunity to discover how to create a new pathway to better cope with life challenges. Like most things that matter in life, there are no real shortcuts. To start the journey to developing coping skills it's helpful to demystify coping.

Perhaps you can relate to Sam; maybe you know someone like him.

Taking charge of one's life starts with awareness and then accepting responsibility for life choices and actions. Each chapter in this book is a building block. The next chapter discusses what mental health is, to facilitate a conversation around the coping crisis and mental health.

CHAPTER 3

Chicken or the Egg

On an early Tuesday morning, Sam is engaged in a process that's disrupting his normal wakeup routine. He typically wakes at 6:00 a.m., gets his coffee and sits at his kitchen table alone, quietly reading the morning paper before taking a shower. This particular morning his mind puts out a radical thought, *Why bother? Just stay in bed for another 30 minutes.*" Taken aback by this automatic thought, Sam wonders why he would not want to read the paper. It's as if he's actively engaged in two conversations happening at the same time. The metaphor of an angel and a devil on his shoulders taking different positions adequately explains what's happening in his head.

Sam is now feeling stressed about the notion of not getting out of bed, as well as the thought of doing what he typically does every morning. He's stuck. What was such a simple decision before now is creating an internal dynamic that's upsetting.

With a little devil on my left shoulder and an angel on my right, both telling me what I should do....
I remind them of the hell you put me through.
The angel falls silent... — Unknown

Sam's depression has been getting heavier over the past month. Even on medication, he has experienced more blue periods and felt a need to sleep more. He's having a hard time getting up the energy to go to work. The weekends have been a write-off; he spends most of the time in bed. The heavy weight of unhappiness this morning is sitting squarely on his head. He gives in and with a slight tear in his eye shakes his head, rolls over and stays in bed for another 30 minutes, knowing that would require him getting on with his day as soon as he woke up, no paper, no quiet time. Sam lets out a big breath, and closes his eyes.

Sam is giving up on one morning activity he has enjoyed for years. What he doesn't know is why. Why this morning is he quitting something he likes and making his world smaller?

The Coping Crisis and Mental Health

Sam now has a serious mental health issue called clinical depression. A person who is experiencing clinical depression often:

- feels helpless and hopeless
- loses interest in daily activities
- engages in self-loathing
- experiences weight changes and sleep challenges
- engages in reckless behaviours to escape the pain of depression
- has difficulty concentrating
- feels irritable
- has thoughts that result in questioning whether life is worth living

Mental Health Risk Continuum

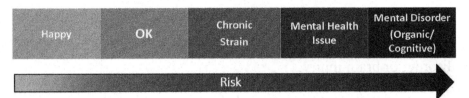

Figure 3-1 — Mental Health Risk Continuum

Mental health is a topic that's gaining attention around the world as a challenge for society and business. Mental health is dynamic; a person can move back and forth on the Mental Health Risk Continuum shown in Figure 3-1, depending on how they are coping with their life stressors.

The progression from happy to mental disorder is meant to display how people typically move along this continuum. In this model it flows from left to right to make the point that it's progressive. Mental health issues often can be linked to a history of cumulative life stressors. A person who has a mental illness has met the criteria for a defined mental disorder that has been given by a trained and accredited professional (e.g., medical doctor, psychologist).

A percentage of mental illness is directly due to genetics, such as issues with neurotransmitters and brain structure. Schizophrenia and bipolar disorder are serious conditions that can benefit from coping skills development, but coping skills alone will not provide the quality of life required to manage these conditions. For this population, professional medical help will define and determine the role and value of psychotropic drugs. A person who develops mental illness due to psychosocial social stressors (e.g., chronic work stress, relationship stress) typically moves through a progression with regard to mental health. Some exceptions that can speed up the onset of a mental illness that are not linked to genetics are serious traumas that can result in post-traumatic stress disorder or brain injury.

Sam was in a coping crisis before he developed his depression. His coping crisis led to his mental health risk that eventually resulted in developing his mental illness issue.

The main thesis of *The Coping Crisis* is that gaps in coping skills are playing a major role in the increase in mental illness. Why these gaps are playing out today is another question. The world has changed and living on a world stage and being plugged in 24-7 is creating a new level of stress.

It would be incorrect to make any inference that gaps in coping skills are the sole cause of mental health issues. Nevertheless, I am confident that gaps in coping skills can explain a significant percentage that makes it worth talking about and promoting the value of developing one's coping skills. If there were fewer people suffering from coping crises there would be fewer people like Sam.

Mental illness can be a by-product of ineffective coping, but it's important again to make it clear I have no intention to suggest that all mental health issues are the result of gaps in coping skills. There's a growing conversation on mental health and its impact. The cumulative cost of providing mental health treatment, care and support services over the next 30 years in Canada is expected to grow to more than $2.5 trillion — that's trillion, not billion.[4] These numbers suggest that with one out of five Canadians suffering from a mental health issue the related costs and risks for business are growing.

Senior business leaders today are more interested in mental health and the potential risk to both employees and employers, but there is much more work to do on this topic. Keep in mind that for the past 100 years we have been talking about physical literacy (e.g., benefits of exercise) and even with all the promotion and focus on physical health that continues today, obesity continues to be a major health problem.

There has been more focus and energy put on mental health. It is starting to get on the radar of senior leaders, who for years have seen the benefits of physical health. As a result, many organizations are funding and supporting employee wellness initiatives such as biometrics, fitness challenges, employee and family assistance programs that provide fitness coaching, and wellness committees that educate the workforce on total health. Even with this focus, employees' overall fitness on average is not improving at the levels most senior leaders would like.

There are lessons that can be taken from employers' efforts to improve physical health literacy that can be applied to curbing mental illness. The first, changing and influencing human behaviour, is challenging and can take much more effort, cost and time than expected. Senior leaders are discovering that the cost of doing nothing to address the growing numbers of employees experiencing stress or mental health issues is mounting.

In Canada, 78 percent of short-term disability claims and 67 percent of long-term claims[5] are due to mental illness. For employers, the stakes are rising, with no major change in sight. By all accounts, mental health problems are predicted to continue to grow. Senior leaders are now asking the *why* question more. As a result, more focus and efforts are being put on curbing mental illness. One early finding, as mentioned earlier, is the role coping skills can play to reduce the chance of a person's psychosocial stressors manifesting into mental health issues, to even becoming a mental illness.

One possible reason why many people are not able to follow through with their physical fitness is due to gaps in their coping skills. Perhaps mental health is a precursor for creating the self-discipline required to take care of one's health. On the surface it appears to make sense if a person is under a great deal of stress and having a hard time coping they may not naturally look or engage in physical activity as a way to cope. For many, physical activity and health require a discipline to create the habits required to integrate this type of activity into their lives on a daily basis. My first degree was in physical education and we taught many years ago the connection between the mind and body. The body depends on a healthy mind just as a healthy mind depends on a healthy body. As a result, there may be a strong agreement to consider the benefits of exercise and physical activity to help a person better cope with their life demands.

Table 3-3 — Beyond Engagement Mental Health Risk Profile[6] has been designed to provide people like Sam with real-time feedback with respect to their current levels of stress, coping, engagement and health. The goal is to help improve employees' awareness, accountability and action to take charge of their

Table 3-3 – **Beyond Engagement Mental Health Risk Profile**

Read the five categories that define the mental health continuum and then take a moment for self-reflection and respond to the following question.
On a typical day, in which category do you spend 85 percent of your time?

Current Mental Health Category	Descriptions for Each Category
Optimal Mental Health	• Presents self in a positive manner • Typically enjoys engaging in pro-social behaviours (exercise, community, etc.) • Energy and drive are evident – presents to the world a positive light • Proven cognitive coping skills to manage and balance the challenges of life and work
Functional Mental Health	• Presents as being content – and, yes, experiences happy moments • Self-disciplined to push through the day – lives life M-T-W-T-F-S-S • Most days has enough energy to get through the day • Able to cope with most days – but often has some script running ……….
Strained Mental Health	• Feels pressure that often releases when changing environments (e.g., leaving work) • Stress is often situational (e.g., peer conflict) and when away from stress can feel OK. Finds it hard being around stressors. • Increased fatigue (mental and physical) • Health habits slip and struggles to cope. Can appear in some situations not as confident as some onlookers would expect.
Challenged Mental Health	• Internally struggling more with internal dialogue to find options that could give some relief • Symptoms starting to chronically have a negative impact on quality of life – happiness and health • Stressful events harder to recover from; often just shuts person down. Symptoms increasing, stress. • May be introduced to psychotropic drugs to cope with anxiety or depression, or sleep medication. • Some may self-medicate as a way to cope with life stress.
Mental Illness (Organic/ Psychosocial)	• Nature vs. nurture: Some folks are born with the generics for a mental health issue, some develop; there is not one road. • Chronic symptoms to be managed, risk for self-harm increasing, risk to others increasing. • It is not uncommon for a person at this level to be medical intervention to help the person manage symptoms (e.g., depression, anxiety). • Has the potential to greatly benefits from development of coping strategies to be able to function at full potential in society.

mental health. How one copes with what are perceived as negative stressors plays an important role in predicting overall ability to live a healthy and fulfilling life.

When stress is not dealt with correctly a person can feel powerless and victimized. Stress attacks the mind and body. The long-term impact of stress is dependent on its frequency, duration and intensity. How a person copes determines how much impact stress has on their mind and body. A coping crisis left without a resolution can lead to a mental health issue.

One key to curb the current coping crisis is for people like Sam to discover they have the final say in how they define and live their life. One critical insight to help a person make this shift is to realize the link between their current thinking and their physical and psychological health. Sam is not aware of how he moved from functional mental health to depression, or how his thinking has influenced his overall physical health.

Sam moved through the mental health continuum, and because he lacked the knowledge and skills to cope, he ultimately was unable to curb his progression from a mental health risk due to chronic work and life stress to developing a mental illness.

Suicide

People like Sam have a high risk profile for suicide. He has all the markers of someone who, if their life does not improve, may reach a point where they no longer want to continue. Forty-nine percent of Canadian male suicide victims fall between the ages of 40 and 64; known as the "hidden epidemic."[7]

The consequences for Sam have been chronic depression and several chronic diseases. One intangible that is impossible to put into words is the degree of hope required for a person to want to keep living. Without hope, a person is at risk for suicide. The candle that burns in each of us can shine brightly or be a light flicker. Sam's candle has not been burning brightly but it's still there or he would have given up by now. Being miserable and wanting to live are two different realities. Sam has felt miserable but wants to live. He had only one moment that tested this decision.

One late Friday night a few years ago Sam had a moment that tested his resolve to live or die. He seldom ever drank; he didn't like the taste and knew he should limit or avoid alcohol while on depression medication. He always followed the rules, so this was no different. For some reason on this night, however, Sam drank a pint of rum with Coke — while sitting outside on the balcony of his apartment. It was a perfect fall evening in

> Why do you think negative mental health issues are on an upward trend?
> What is happening?

early October. He was looking out at the clear night, lit up by bright stars and a full harvest moon.

Since Sam seldom drinks he had no tolerance for the rum. Within 20 minutes of finishing the bottle the alcohol hit him like a brick. He was now under the influence and experienced a feeling he had never experienced before. His mind was racing all over the place. His lens of the world changed and he started to see and think a bit differently in this drunken state. His unconscious mind went to work on him and started to attack him for being a weak human being.

Sam's unconscious mind started generating automatic thoughts: *drink?* "Why has it taken so long to let go, relax and enjoy a drink? Why am I so tense? Why sit here alone? Why is life so hard? Don't be a loser anymore; this is exactly what's needed to have fun. Let go and go to a bar. Time to find a woman. Stop being alone."

Sam's unconscious mind went on and on for an hour without mercy, but he resisted all its commands to take action. His fear of getting into trouble took over and his practical side kicked in and stopped his unconscious mind, which took this decision and changed its tactic. "Fine, no fun. Perfect. Alone again. So what's the purpose of living if there's no joy? No one cares; just end it. Real peace will not happen until death." This message got into Sam's conscious mind and he started to agree with this logic. He ran the story of all his pain and regret. The feelings associated with this came to the surface hard and fast. He was now feeling terrible with grief, anger and depression all at the same time.

Sam was starting to navigate a life or death decision that I call the "utopia decision." It's the conversation as to why living or dying makes sense. It's all based on hope. When hope is lost comes powerful cognitive dissonance that rationalizes within the conscious brain the value and benefits of dying, and the best course is to bring this life to a peaceful ending. This is not always the case. Some people, due to a situational stressor, decide in the moment to kill themselves. The means of dying is often violent: shooting or hanging, or it can be passive, such as taking pills. The person picks a strategy they can cope with so they can perform the act.

The utopia decision is different. A person can make a decision to end their life and live normally for two weeks. The choice of death is perceived to be easy, like jumping, where the act does the work versus the person. There's little planning required, just picking the spot. What's so important for a person who is caught in this decision is to know that it's blinding, like a trance. There's always hope, but in this state no hope will come unless it's from the outside or the person is stopped, comes out of the trance, and realizes they do want to live.

It's normal, under significant stress, to have an automatic thought that suggests suicide as an option. The conscious brain typically dismisses this quickly. This thought doesn't mean one is suicidal; it means their creative system is actively looking for a solution. Under the influence of alcohol, Sam's conscious mind started to consider the unconscious mind's suggestions. He allowed his mind to consider suicide as a viable option and thought about the benefits of no more stress, no more manager, no more regret, no more feeling alone, etc. When he thought about how he would do it his conscious brain turned back on strong and shut down this line of thinking. Sam was not a confident person and the thought of killing himself was scary. This fear helped to snap him back and stop this line of thinking. He was shaken that he had allowed his mind to go as far as it did.

Thinking about suicide is one thing. Fortunately, typically there is often a significant gap between thinking about suicide and acting on it. When a person starts to make a plan, gets the means to carry it out and sets a time and place, the risk increases as the gap is closed. At this point, the utopia decision mode starts to become more locked in. It's common for a person in this mode to carry on for days or even weeks without anyone knowing anything is wrong and out of the blue it seems to onlookers that the person just suddenly took their own life.

What the average person may not know is that losing hope is a utopia decision. Once the light goes out the person sees deciding to end their life as the best way to cope. At this stage, all hope or any chance that things could have been better has been lost. The decision is not rational; it's based on the person's conscious brain giving up on hope. Their candle has gone out and the future has only darkness and pain, and suicide to them is really a wonderful option to finding peace. Again, not a rational decision but how the mind smoothes the edges. Unless the person is found out and an intervention happens to create a spark for hope they are on automatic pilot, taking the steps they have agreed to in their utopia decision until their last moment alive.

Living or dying is each person's ultimate decision. Coping plays a role in determining how far a person under stress will go to find peace and how much hope they can maintain. A person has to see something that is of value to keep them going. It can be hope, a pet, friends, work, family or self-acceptance. It doesn't

The benefits of improved coping skills extend beyond the potential for better prevention and care of mental health challenges. For the Sams who work in environments where risk of bodily injury is high, developing good coping skills may well prove very beneficial in the prevention of serious injuries in the workplace.
~Conrad Ferguson, Partner, Morneau Shepell

matter. It only matters at that moment to find something that means something. In this moment, Sam picked himself. His conscious mind perhaps saw some positive in his life. He has a job and money.

This was the only time Sam drank to this point. It was also the only time he thought about hurting himself. This was his last time for drinking and he's not had another moment since like this one. He still lives with daily stress, and without a resolution this dark October night may return.

It's beneficial for a person like Sam to gain insight into why and how coping skills play a role in influencing their mental health risk. Before it evolves into a mental illness, mental health risk can act like the flu. A person can feel sick and have tough moments, and then over a period of time start to feel better when the stress is stopped. The cure for people like Sam starts by becoming aware of things that can be done to better manage external and internal stressors. Like the flu, when neglected, mental health risk can become very serious, even terminal.

Employers Can Help

Employers can take actions to remove and reduce environmental stressors and hazards, such as making a commitment to eliminate workplace bullying, harassment and unnecessary red tape. They can appoint trained and skilled managers and focus on building integrated employee engagement, mental health and respectful workplace strategies.

Employee and family assistance programs and coping skills developmental programs facilitate coping skills that reduce employee risk and help to maximize productivity. But this action alone will not do it. Success is dependent on each employee taking accountability and being open and motivated to develop their coping skills. Employees are more likely to opt in when they are clear on the value proposition and benefits to them directly. The good news is coping skills help them both at work and at home. Most employees struggling to cope benefit from coping skills training. Coping often takes time to learn because it deals with emotions, beliefs, needs, wants, expectations and environmental stressors.

What comes first, a coping crisis or mental illness? For a person who doesn't have a genetic mental illness I believe it's a coping crisis. The mental health continuum provides a visual overview of how a person can move back and forth on the scale based on how they are dealing with stress demands and how long those demands are present. Sometimes situations change and the stress can appear to be gone, until the next wave.

When a person like Sam, who has no organic mental health issues, gets caught in a coping crisis they are at risk of developing a mental health issue if they do not get relief from the stress they are

> So what comes first, mental health issues or poor coping skills?

experiencing. Society has evolved to help such people through what is known as talk therapy. Leading cognitive theorists have shown the world through years of clinical practice that talk therapy can help a person change their life and learn to make better choices.[8] This therapy facilitates and develops one's coping skills. I would argue the point based on my research that there is a strong relationship between a person's coping skills and their risk for mental health issues.

If someone doesn't ask for nor accept help they can remain stuck, just like Sam, who has yet to consider or explore therapy, even after his doctor suggested it as an option. He doesn't believe talking about his life or his choices could possibly make things better. He's creating the rules for his life with this type of thinking, and these rules are limiting his potential, as evidenced by his current situation and health.

Another reality is people like Sam may not even know they need help. Employees whose employers provide them an opportunity to self-evaluate their coping skills, health and lifestyle habits are in a better position to ask for help. Employers who also provide coping skills training and an opportunity for an employee like Sam to develop new skills may end up helping the Sams of the world that don't even realize how at risk they are and the value of this guidance to help transform lifestyle choice, health and overall quality of life at work and home. It is my assertion for people who have no organic mental health risk factors (e.g., genetically predisposed for bipolar, etc.), who are facing a coping crisis, that this is one key indicator of a person's risk for mental health issues that can become a mental illness (such as addictive disorders, depression and anxiety).

The next chapter introduces five life challenges that can create stress when they are not fulfilled.

CHAPTER 4

Five Life Challenges

Sam gets out of bed, once again starting his day off feeling frustrated. For all the hours he has spent thinking about his life he has not made any significant improvements. He takes his shower, gets ready and begins his short drive to work. He once again ponders, "Why is my life so hard; why can't it be easier?" This is a common question asked by people struggling to cope with the various challenges life presents.

Five common life challenges that influence the average person's overall perception of their current life satisfaction are money, career, relationship, self-esteem and health. Each of these can be a source of stress.

Sam goes to work each day feeling helpless. He quietly feels he's trapped and he sees little hope that things will be better. Learned helplessness is a psychological state involving a disturbance of motivation, cognitive processes and emotionality as a result of previously experienced failure.[9] For reasons he may not fully understand, Sam has taken the position that he will adhere to his manager's requests, demands and instructions without any resistance or question. As a result, Sam's thinking negatively impacts his self-esteem, cognitive flexibility and creativity. This helpless state and his lack of coping skills have resulted in his weakened emotional state, which has led to depression.

Table 4-1 provides an overview of five life challenges that every human being will face in their lifetime. Imagine if Sam had only 10 brain units each day to focus on the five life challenges. Where he spends his focus and energy can have an impact on his overall life satisfaction and health. Sam spends all 10 of his brain units on money and career, so he has none left to spend on relationships, self or health.

Stepping back and looking at Sam's overall psychological and physical health, it's not a surprise that he has so many issues. When a person is in a coping crisis they tend to focus on stressors and look for ways to cope with them. The way in which Sam copes is clearly not in his long-term best health interests.

Not based on any pure science but simply anecdotal feedback from thousands of workshop participants taking a course from me on a variety of topics from health and wellness, stress management to coping, the average person spends eight brain units on money, career and relationships. This does not leave much energy for self-acceptance and health. There appears to be a correlation between this statistic and why many people have poor health, as they have not made their health a priority. It is helpful to become aware of where one spends one's effort daily, and the consequenc-

Insanity: doing the same thing over and over again and expecting different results. — Albert Einstein

Table 4-1 — The Five Life Challenges

Money	To obtain enough money to achieve the lifestyle one defines as acceptable. Setting realistic expectations and living within one's means is critical for money management. To do so requires having a simple budget that monitors money in and out. Financial stability requires focus to manage debt, cash flow, and retirement.
Career	The majority of human beings are not born into money. As a result, they are dependent on work to pay for their lifestyle. A job whose sole purpose is to make money to pay bills will rarely ever be fulfilling. Individuals who are in careers where they enjoy going to work every day, believe that what they do is important, and take pride in their work are likely to feel productive and fulfilled.
Relation-ships	Every healthy human being benefits from and desires caring, healthy, and loving relationships. There are different kinds of relationships: casual, professional, and intimate. Most people want and expect to have safe and healthy relationships in each of the three categories. Developing relationships takes time and energy.
Self-Acceptance	Looking into the mirror and liking what one sees inside and out is required for self-acceptance, which influences self-esteem and belief in an individual's ability to achieve their life goals and desires. What a person thinks about themselves influences what they believe they can do. Coping skills are tools that a person can use to solve life challenges. However, coping skills include one's self-efficacy, the belief in their ability to achieve a defined outcome.
Health	From the day a human being is born they are on a journey that has a defined timeline and ending. What a person does daily with respect to their pro-health choices influences their mental and physical health. Yes, there are genetic factors that must be ruled in. However, lifestyle and healthy habits play an important role in preventing disease. Health requires discipline and attention. Exercise, nutrition, sleep, and relaxation are key elements for promoting health.

es and benefits. For Sam the consequences are evident, but the benefits not so much.

It is quite common for the average person to have several conflicting priorities that put demands on their energy and time. Because of the constant pull and demands, mental health and/or physical health is often not made a priority. One key step to creating a better balance of these five categories is <u>awareness</u> where one is spending their energy and then taking <u>accountability</u> for one's choices to take <u>action</u> to meet unmet needs. The AAA approach can help reset and refocus one's approach to life.

One helpful AAA activity is to pick one area that you want to focus and improve upon in the next 90 days. Be clear on why you want to improve. Once you do this the next step is to track the number of brain units you are spending on each category on a daily basis (remember for this activity your total needs to add to 10), and then chart your daily results. Once you put your results down ask yourself what you can do better the next day. It is rare a person who does this exercise for 90 days who will not have some benefit and start to take even more action in the areas they choose to improve. Why? Because if one is motivated to do this exercise they are also typically motivated to change and do the work to re-align priorities and energy. If you struggle with this activity and cannot find the answers this may be a good time to explore your options to find new perspectives. What is important to know is you would not be alone, and asking for help is OK. These five life challenges are where most life stressors are generated.

Sam trusts his work skills; it's his coping skills that have let him down. To be fair, he never learned how to cope better with people or work. He never had a mentor, never had a coach, and never took coping skills training. Like many people, Sam is caught in a coping skills crisis that has moved him from mental health issues to developing depression. He's unaware how he became depressed and that there are any options for him to get out of it. He certainly feels trapped. He's not aware that he's getting sicker as each year passes, and he won't get better unless he does something different.

For Sam to make a shift he will benefit from spending brain units on relationships, self-esteem and health. To do so he will first need to learn how to curb the current stress load he faces each day. When he can better cope with stress he will be in a better position to learn how to cope better with his life.

The next chapter provides a review of stress with respect to how stress impacts the mind and body.

CHAPTER 5

The Fuel

The fuel that drives a coping crisis is an individual's perception of their world. Neuroscience teaches that the mind is constantly interacting with the world through billions of chemical interactions that facilitate how the brain defines its reality. There's a notion in neuroscience that suggests each person is making up their reality as they go.[10] As a result, no two people see or experience the same situation the exact same way. This can result in frustration and stress in human interactions. One of the principal causes of stress for human beings is relationship conflict.

Sam's ultimate health and happiness are dependent on how well he interacts with his external and internal worlds. Having a difference between what one wants and has creates what we typically define as stress.

There are two kinds of stress: 1) good stress (eustress) and, 2) unhealthy stress (distress). Stress in moderation can be positive and can help motivate human behaviour to achieve a desired outcome.

From this point on, when using the word stress it will be referring to distress and how it can have a negative impact on health. Typically associated with distress are painful emotions such as rejection and failure. Stress, if allowed to grow, can lead to permanent structural change to the body's health (e.g., heart disease). Stress can kill because of the way it attacks the mind and body. It can be difficult for the layperson to understand how the body's protection system, which was designed to protect, can also attack.

Human beings typically do not like pain and want it to stop as fast as possible. Any action to stop pain may not necessarily get to the root cause; it may just be a Band-Aid. At the core of many mental health issues is a person's inability to align resources to figure out how to cope with their life in a healthy and productive way. As a result, they end up becoming overwhelmed by life stressors, which can have a negative impact on their overall mental health.

Stress is a term for which there is no universally accepted definition, though it's clear that most of the population knows bad stress is something they don't want. Stress is the fuel that drives many mental health issues and chronic disease.

Understanding how stress attacks the mind or body in some cases can help motivate people like Sam. It also can help them understand why developing coping skills can be challenging when under stress.

The intensity to which a person can experience stress falls on a scale from mild to severe. The more intense the stressor, the more distracting and all-consuming the stress will be. Most stress falls within three categories:

- **Acute stress** — Stress that arises from day-to-day interaction in the world that is due to some kind of conflict that is often temporary

- **Chronic stress (subordinate stress)** — The result of an acute stressor such as a work-related issue that goes on day in and day out (e.g., conflict with your boss) that wears at the person daily and puts them at risk for suffering the negative impacts of stress, such as stress-related illness

- **Traumatic stress** — A stressor that is outside a person's normal coping skills, such as an accident or disaster. Researchers have estimated that 75 percent of all people experience some form of trauma in life: the loss or suffering of a loved one, the diagnosis of an illness, the pain of divorce or separation, the shock of an accident, assault or disaster. Estimates suggest that around 20 percent of all people are likely to experience a potentially traumatic event within a given year.[11]

Each type of stress can create its own set of challenges. For example, traumatic stress can lead to post-traumatic stress disorder. One intense experience, if not dealt with properly, can lead to a lifetime of burden. To understand the impact of stress there's a benefit to developing insight into the role of the body's protection system and the risks associated when this system is overly active.

Fight-or-Flight Response

There are two systems that provide important information as to how stress can impact the mind and body. The first is the *fight-or-*

flight system, which is immediate and happens in real time. When it turns on, it is clear to the person there is something happening. The second is the general adaptation syndrome (see below), which may not be as obvious to a person, but when allowed to happen over an extended period of time can have a negative impact on a person's overall health. Both put chemicals into the body that, when not needed, over time can have a negative impact. The purpose of this section is to provide a brief summary of how these two systems work.

When a person is overwhelmed by external stimuli and can't get their psychological bearing as to what to do and the degree of threat, it's normal for the body to automatically start to make physiological changes, with the goal of protecting itself. This onboard operating system that turns on automatically is referred to as the *fight-or-flight* response.

When one is exposed to a perceived or real threat, it triggers in the operating system that a threat or danger is present — take action now. This action is hardwired into the human brain; there's no turning it half on or off. Once it turns on, it's on. Its purpose is to fight or flee from danger. Unfortunately, the system doesn't differentiate between real and perceived threats. Since its sole function is to protect the body it's constantly in a ready-set-go mode and monitoring the external world looking for threats. When this system turns on it changes the person's physiological state to prepare the body to take action.

The *fight-or-flight* response evolved to assist human beings to move from being the hunted to the hunter. Our ability to process fear was critical for our survival. Eventually, we ended up at the top of the food chain. Today, the *fight-or-flight* response is often overkill. For example, the response is not designed to tell the difference or process the discrepancy between a bear and an upset co-worker. When the body becomes threatened (real or perceived) it reacts. The logic of what gets one person upset is often dependent on how well they can manage their emotions under pressure.

During stressful conditions, the activity of the sympathetic nervous system increases to prepare the body for the *fight-or-flight* response. The adrenal gland's first reaction is to send epinephrine (adrenaline) into the bloodstream, which directly impacts the body (e.g., speeds up heart rate). In addition, the adrenal gland puts out more cortisol and other kinds of glucocorticoids that turn sugar in the body into energy.

Finally, the last biggest chemical released from nerve cells is norepinephrine, whose purpose is to prepare the five senses and muscles for action, making them ready for fight or flight. Norepinephrine is released from the adrenal medulla (the core of the adrenal glands). Neurotransmitters are powerful hormones that are secreted by the brain and nervous system and have a powerful effect on our psychological and physical health. How the body responds when the *fight-or-flight* system is turned on:

- Stored sugars and fats are released into the bloodstream to provide quick energy.

- Breathing quickens to provide more oxygen to the blood.

- Muscles tense in preparation for action.

- Digestion ceases so that more blood is available to the brain and muscles.

- Blood-clotting mechanisms are activated to protect against possible injury.

- Perspiration increases to help reduce body temperature.

- The pupils dilate and the sense of smell and hearing become more acute.

- Increased heart rate, blood pressure and respiration, pumping more blood to the muscles, supplying more oxygen to the muscles and heart-lung system.

- Thickening of the blood — to increase oxygen supply (red cells), enabling better defence from infections (white cells) and to stop bleeding quickly (platelets).

- Prioritizing — increased blood supply to peripheral muscles and heart, to motor and basic-functions regions in the brain; decreased blood supply to digestive system and irrelevant brain regions (such as speech areas). This also causes secretion of body wastes, leaving the body lighter.

- Secretion of adrenaline and other stress hormones — to further increase the response, and to strengthen relevant systems.

- Secretion of endorphins — natural painkillers, providing an instant defense against pain.

- The stress response hormones cause a number of biochemical and physiological changes.

Regardless of why the *fight-or-flight* is turned on, it works the same. A series of chemical reactions that collectively prepare the body to fight (take a stand) or flee (get to safety) is launched. The *fight-or-flight* response supports the person's decision to take a stand and fight or to turn and run from a situation.

One risk with the *fight-or-flight* system occurs when it stays on for extended periods or is overly activated. Both result in a continuous release of chemicals and hormones. If these chemicals continue to enter the body when it is not in real physical danger and doesn't need to use them to survive, they become toxic to the body and start to break down its natural defence systems, because the body is constantly releasing cortisol.

A not-so-obvious problem of stress is that when the *fight-or-flight* response is activated it turns off the body's immune system, like a power grid system would do to reroute energy. As a result, a person under chronic strain has a weakened immune system, which puts them at more risk for becoming ill and catching common illnesses like colds and flu.

The *fight-or-flight* response can be triggered from the external world as well as the internal world. For example, the jealous partner who overreacts to a situation without any evidence. In this case, an automatic thought fires off powerful emotions of doubt that create images of a partner cheating. The conscious brain accepts this notion without the facts and acts by blaming or accusing the partner of cheating. This automatic thinking driven by emotion can end up destroying a relationship because one partner could not control their emotions and overreacted, creating psychological damage to the relationship and now one partner does not think the other is safe to be around and they become wired as a threat. This is a real-life example where coping skills could create a different and better outcome.

When we are awake, the brain is constantly monitoring the environment (unconsciously and consciously) for threats and opportunities. Much of the activity and automatic thoughts a person creates come from their unconscious mind. For example, when someone cuts you off at an intersection the thoughts that come to your mind are often automatic. For some, this trigger of emotion can result in road rage. The unconscious brain provides the conscious mind unfiltered ideas because it has no filter with respect to good or bad. As a result, ideas that are generated unconsciously may not be in a person's best interest. Luckily, the conscious brain is hard at work judging what is good or bad for the person to help determine what ideas make sense to act on. Coping skills influence what a person rationalizes as good or bad.

The unconscious brain has the ability to launch powerful emotions that can erupt to the surface like a volcano. There's lots of heat with these intense emotions (e.g., fear, rage). They demand an immediate reaction by the conscious brain to do something. Emotions can lead a person's behavioural system until the conscious mind catches up and takes control. Emotions unchecked will overrule the logical, conscious brain. For a person like Sam with low coping skills it seems impossible to control emotions, especially powerful ones like love, grief, jealousy, fear, hate, anger and rage.

A person's coping skills define their ability to dampen emotions associated with stressful interactions, as well as manage their choices at a conscious level. Thoughts charged with intense emotion influence behaviour if the conscious mind does not influence picking healthy versus unhealthy choices to actions. Consider the person being cut off at an intersection generating the random thought, "Just smash my car into the back of this bugger that just cut me off. This will teach them not to mess with me." The mind works fast and as a result the conscious brain has its hands full to manage the unconscious mind creatively. Often, the conscious mind can dismiss a random thought quickly. The challenge for some is when the mind starts to debate what is good or bad. A person with low coping skills is more at risk to give in to bad choices and put themselves at more risk in the moment if over a period of time the behaviour is repeated, like Sam's nightly eating.

Possibly because of the constant debates between the conscious and unconscious mind this can partially explain why some people blame their environment for their decisions. The unconscious mind creates only automatic thoughts; it doesn't evaluate the risk, source or impact of the thought. This is the conscious mind's job. Possibly, because the power of emotions is why Sam is struggling to accept his choices are made from within and are not defined by the outside world. Through this lens, this may be why Sam is stressed out and frustrated, why he blames his environment, and spends energy rationalizing his position as having no choice or control over his own life.

All life is an experiment. The more experiments you make the better. —
Ralph Waldo Emerson

General Adaptation Syndrome

The general adaptation syndrome (GAS) is not as dramatic as the *fight-or-flight* system, but it explains how the body can break down when confronted with chronic stress on a daily basis. If ignored, like the *fight-or-flight* system, it will have a negative impact on one's long-term health. The GAS explains how stress impacts the body[12] daily on a chronic basis. The frequency, duration and intensity in which a person is engaged in this model define its impact on their short- and long-term health. Following is an overview of the model's three stages:

Stage 1: Alarm Phase — The body starts out in a neutral state of being unstressed. But once stress starts to intrude on the person, such as someone taking their parking spot, a stressor develops. Each stressor impacts the body as an alarm. The purpose of the alarm stage is to prepare to protect and defend the body, which starts to become aroused and activates the sympathetic nervous system, releasing hormones to prepare to activate the *fight-or-flight* response. Throughout the day, each person is exposed to a variety of perceived stressors in their work environment that can increase their level of stress (e.g., conflicts with a peer, client or a manager). In this stage the body's chemistry changes due to stress: 1) temperature and blood pressure drop; 2) heart rate quickens; and 3) muscles become weakened with excessive hormones. The body can't maintain such a heightened degree of arousal for long, so it moves to the next phase if the stress is not resolved.

Stage II: Resistance Phase — Most stressful situations are not severe enough to cause death, which allows the person to enter the resistance phase. This is the body's attempt to survive in an aroused state and adjust to the stressors of the environment. In this phase, the body is trying to compensate and adapt to the stressors. Its physiology has been elevated to the maximum level of stress where the individual is still organically alive and functioning. Though the person is still functioning, it's important to note that their cognitive abilities are decreased, which can impact decision-making abilities.

The body makes the following kinds of compensations. The pituitary gland releases adrenocorticotropic hormones and stimulates the adrenal cortex to continue releasing cortico-steroids. This hormone works to increase the body's resistance to stress. As resistance to specific stressors increases, most of the physiological processes return to normal. Although things appear normal, they are not. To survive in this phase, the body is forced to use a large amount of its energy stores (minerals, sugar and hormones). It reacts as though it is in a low-grade, chronic level of *fight-or-flight*, and will, over time, expose the person to the potential of stress-related illness that can result in chronic disease. Once

---

Over my 30-year career as an occupational health nurse, I have met many people who had to take time off work or long-term disability leave due to stress, anxiety and depression. Some have made suicide attempts.

We live in an era of great change and transformation, and where coping skills are essential to all of us and imperatives for organizational survival. It is necessary that a book like The Coping Crisis written by Dr. Bill Howatt be read by as many people as possible.

~Claudine Ducharme, Partner, National Health Consulting at Morneau Shepell and Professional Coach

again, the person can't stay in this phase for long before the body will start to break down.

Stage III: Exhaustion Phase — With continued exposure to chronic stress, which is perceived as bad by the person, over a period of time, the body's ability to resist stress weakens, until there is a physiological collapse. This is the beginning of the exhaustion phase. The pituitary gland and adrenal cortex are unable to continue secreting their hormones, and the person is unable to keep up their energy levels to fight stress. The body is no longer able to produce adrenalin, because blood sugar levels have declined. The person has little ability to tolerate stress, and will report being mentally and physically tired.

When the body is at a chronic level of stress, it's similar to the gas pedal on a car being stuck. The body keeps producing gas (chemicals) even after the threat or stressor is gone. This is where the hypothalamus-pituitary-adrenal axis (critical component of the human endocrine system) is locked on. This overactive axis produces more chemicals than the body needs, and if not turned off will eventually lead to a decrease in production of interleukin-6, an immune-system messenger. In this phase, a person has a compromised immune system and is at greater risk of stress illness.

It's a commonly accepted conclusion in the medical world that chronic psychological stress over an extended period of time

What keeps me going is goals. — Muhammad Ali

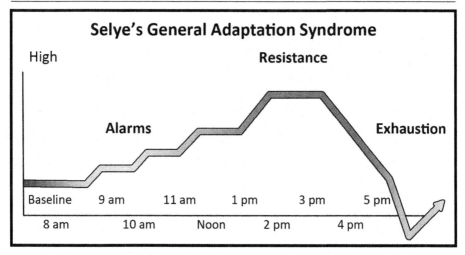

Figure 5-1 — General Adaptation Syndrome

can put a person at risk for developing psychological and/or physical health issues. Sam has heard from his doctor the benefits of being properly hydrated, eating nutritious food, and engaging in physical activity such as exercise and outdoor recreation to burn off the toxic chemicals he builds up through the day. His doctor knows that if Sam could shift his focus at the end of the day and engage in an activity like exercise and learn to like it this would be one positive step to take better control of his overall health. But this doesn't get to the root cause of the stress nor how to cope with it.

Figure 5-1 maps out a typical day of the different alarms that challenge Sam's physiology. They can be minor, from someone moving his favourite mug, to interactions with his manager. Each person has different tolerance levels. It's common for a person with high levels of stress to have low tolerance levels.

As the day proceeds, Sam's mind and body can no longer fight off the daily grind of stress and his body naturally follows a pattern where it starts to crash, as it can no longer resist the environment. As a result, when Sam's day is over at 7:00 p.m., he's mentally and physically spent and ready for a break.

Stress is not just hard on one's emotions and thinking. It's hard on the body at the chemical level. Becoming aware of how one reacts to stress is an important step in learning how to manage it better. This is often a first step for taking responsibility for one's behaviour.

Stress Outcomes

Frustration is a common symptom when a person perceives they are under pressure and stress. Frustration is an intense emotion that if not controlled has the potential to become aggression and anger. When a person is frustrated they try to regain a sense of control to eliminate the causes of their stress and frustration.[13] When their stress levels are high they typically have a lower frustration tolerance. This means it takes little stress or pressure to feel overwhelmed. People with a low frustration tolerance often develop what is known as irrational beliefs (thinking)[14] that create a set of internal rules as to how things should be and why it makes sense for them to feel the way they do. For example, Sam believes he should never speak his mind or he will get fired. He has no evidence that this is true; it's just what he believes. He has created this rule. As a result, he has trapped himself in a position where he will not share his thinking when he believes it may create any debate with his manager.

Sam's current lack of coping skills has resulted in feeling like each day he's running a mini-marathon. He's sick, and the longer he stays in this stress cycle, the higher the risk that he will get sicker. He's paying a high price by not learning to cope better with his stress. Since he perceives his stress is greater than his resources, it's not only having a negative impact on his cognitive abilities with respect to his perception whether or not he can cope with work, it's also affecting his physiology.

Once Sam gets home he's mentally and physically exhausted. The further he goes below the baseline (see figure 5-1), the longer it will take him to recover. He has developed an unhealthy set of habits that are hindering him from getting back to baseline: he stays alone for hours in front of the TV and mindlessly eats. This sedentary lifestyle has facilitated his chronic illnesses, but he has not yet connected all the dots.

One risk for Sam is that if he continues on this cycle he can develop burnout. Burnout is a state of physical, emotional and mental exhaustion as well as a syndrome of emotional exhaustion, depersonalization of others, and a feeling of reduced personal accomplishment.[15]

Edelwich and Brodsky have delineated four stages (see Figure 5-2) that burnout is likely to go through. When a person gets to stage 4 this represents a serious mental health challenge. Burnout is associated with workplace stress and demand on a person's perceptions of their current resources. Coping skills can help reduce the risk for moving up this continuum.

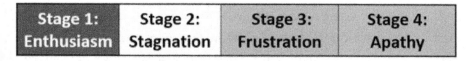

Stage 1: Enthusiasm	Stage 2: Stagnation	Stage 3: Frustration	Stage 4: Apathy

Figure 5-2 — Burnout Continuum

Stage 1: Enthusiasm — The individual enters their job with high hopes and perhaps even unrealistic expectations. However, they are positive and motivated to do their best work.

Stage 2: Stagnation — The worker starts to feel that personal, financial and career needs are not being met. Sometimes it may seem that less-able colleagues are moving faster up the career ladder. If intrinsic and extrinsic reinforcement does not occur, the worker will move to the next stage of burnout.

Stage 3: Frustration — The worker is in trouble. They begin to question efforts put forth as to their effectiveness, value and impact in the face of ever-mounting obstacles. As burnout is contagious, it's necessary that the worker be directly confronted by arranging workshops or support groups to increase awareness of the burnout syndrome and generate problem solving as a group. These efforts may lead the way back to a tempered form of enthusiasm or, if not effective, the final stage of burnout.

Stage 4: Apathy — is the chronic indifference to the situation. At this stage the individual is in a state of disequilibrium (inability to control emotions or cognitions) and immobility (inability to behave up to their potential due to being in a state of stress). They will also likely be in a state of denial and have little objective understanding of what is occurring. Therapy is necessary for reversal to take place.

When you have come to the edge of all the light you have. And step into the darkness of the unknown. Believe that one of the two will happen to you. Either you'll find something solid to stand on. Or you'll be taught how to fly. — Richard Bachi

Sam has been moving back and forth between stage 2 (stagnation) and stage 3 (frustration) for the past few years. His work skills and IT capabilities get him through. He loves his work, just not the grind, but he is questioning how long he can continue the pace. Sam's body and mind have broken down already and if he stays in this cycle much longer he could move to stage 4 (apathy) and lose the joy in his work. He would then be at risk for believing he really has nothing left. His resolve to go to work remains in place and keeps him going, as painful as it is. He has created what he may believe is a safe sanctuary: being in front of his TV, which paradoxically is really a disease chamber.

Sam is not alone. It's not uncommon for people to develop unhealthy coping strategies such as drugs, alcohol, anger and overeating in order to overcome negative emotions to feel better. Stress is not objective. Each person has their own filter that defines what is and is not stressful. The environment gives information but in the end each person defines what they can and cannot cope with. Again, it doesn't matter if stress is real or perceived; both can have a negative impact on the body.

Stress is dealt with via two kinds of actions: 1) problem-focused coping — controls the stressful situation directly; 2) emotion-focused coping — control of one's emotions in the stressful situation.[16] A person can attempt to do both, but normally will put their resources into one of the two possibilities.

Luke: All right, I'll give it a try.
Yoda: No. Try not. Do . . . Or do not. There is no try.

In Sam's case, he's been dealing with controlling his emotions. His conscious brain has decided there are no alternatives. He's still unaware of how his emotions are influencing his brain chemistry and how this is impacting his thinking and overall health. People typically perceive the root cause of their stress as being driven by environmental stressors (e.g., noise and air pollution) and social stressors (peer pressure and a negative workplace).

Everyone will be faced with stress sometime in their life; there's no escaping it. In the end, it's not the amount of stress that determines a person's stress level; it's how they are able to process and cope with stress cognitively.[17]   The better a person can manage their psychological state, the less negative impact stress will have on their immune system, which protects the body from illness, disease and mental health issues.

The challenge with stress is the cognitive energy it takes. As stress fires off emotions, the old brain gives a clear direction of what it thinks the person needs to do. Sam's old brain, for example, told him to quit more than one thing in life, which has resulted in his current social network and lifestyle.

This decision to quit has provided no relief. Sam spends hours thinking about how unhappy he is and rationalizes why he needs to stay where he is and why he's stuck there. This loop has gone on for years and nothing has changed for the good. With no resolution or peace, the same old thoughts, feelings and behaviours keep replaying themselves.

Human thinking errors can prolong and create stress. The mind is capable of processing vast amounts of information, but with all the billions of chemical interactions that are involved in filtering the information we see, hear and learn, the possibility for error is high.

When facing stress there is value in accepting the notion that it's possible that some automatic thoughts may be wrong. An effective coping approach is to slow down and get the best available facts, establish the root cause, explore available resources, and make a decision that may help reduce the number of thinking errors one will make.

No two people filter external stressors in the same manner; what is stressful for one person may not be to another. There are two actions when a person is faced with stress: primary appraisal (what is the potential threat?) and secondary appraisal (once the individual knows what it is, they must determine what they can do to cope).[17] At this point, when a person is assessing whether they can cope with a stress event they are also assessing its impact:

- **Harm/Loss** — impact of damage that has occurred (e.g., fired from job)

- **Threat** — potential for a particular harm or loss (e.g., potential cutbacks)

- **Challenge** — opportunity for personal and emotional gain; however, the person must muster all their physical and psychological energy to succeed in this challenge

Depending on the person's coping skills, the impact and stakes influence the level of risk they are willing to take.

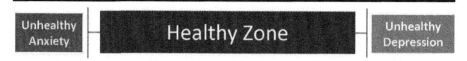

Figure 5-3 - Healthy Zone Continuum

It's common for a person when engaged in a stress-strain relationship (e.g., work stress that results in developing a headache) for their stress to evolve if they don't get relief. How a person copes with stress can be demonstrated in Figure 5-3 — Healthy Zone Continuum. Depression and anxiety are common at low levels under pressure and can fall within the normal zone range. Each person under pressure gravitates to one end or the other — anxiety or depression. When the stress continues it's possible for anxiety and depression to move outside the normal zone. This is when the symptoms associated with depression and anxiety can start to become problematic. When a person starts to experience such symptoms it's common for them to become concerned and distracted by this change in their mental health.

Stress symptoms like depression and anxiety are normal ways for the mind and body to cope, but these alone do not mean a person has a mental health issue. What defines the risk for a mental health issue are the frequency, duration and intensity of these symptoms and their impact on the person's overall quality of life.

People who use anger to cope do so in an attempt to take control of their situation. There are three kinds of aggression[18]:

- Displaced aggression, when a person does not feel confident or safe to deal directly with their source of frustration (e.g., manager) and redirects their frustration to another (e.g., takes it out at home with their spouse).

- Direct aggression, when a person directs their aggression directly to the person they are frustrated with and has the potential to escalate to anger.

- Withdrawing or escaping aggression, when a person takes steps to withdraw or escape a situation to deal with stress.

The example cited above provides evidence that with stress, frustration and aggression come inter-relationship conflict. There are also three common ways a person will cope with inter-relationship conflict[19]:

- **Approach-approach conflict** — This occurs when a person has the choice between two alternatives that regardless of the choice the consequences are going to be pleasurable.

- **Avoidance-avoidance conflict** — This is the opposite of approach-approach conflict. In this situation, both choices will lead to an unwanted sequence.

- **Approach-avoidance conflict** — This situation is challenging and complicated because in this kind of conflict there is an opportunity for both a pleasurable and unwanted consequence.

Sam doesn't feel comfortable with conflict. Many like him avoid conflict; it's often viewed as a negative. People confident with their coping skills who engage in conflict have an opportunity to learn and grow. Conflict has the potential to facilitate new learnings. Those who never develop coping skills to deal with conflict are at risk for building up unresolved conflict, which can eat at them. Sam has unresolved conflict with his manager, meaning he has issues with him. This conflict is fuelling stress for Sam but his manager doesn't know about this. If Sam doesn't develop coping skills or deal with the conflict it will grow and continue to do damage to his happiness and health.

Another risk for prolonged stress is the increase of counter-productive behaviours. There's a wide range of such behaviours, from being late for work, to lying to a manager, to bursts of anger. These actions do not always mean a person is bad; they can be associated with negative coping skills. In the corporate workplace, these kinds of behaviours can decrease productivity and risk people's safety. Besides this obvious risk of hurting others, anger can lead to chronic stress that can cause illness, and even homicide or suicide. The stakes are high. Coping skills are important for protecting a person from themselves, as well as protecting others.

The next chapter introduces a concept called coping churn. This provides insight into how people like Sam often think themselves into situations. Stress is the fuel that feeds coping churn, which is the engine that drives a coping crisis.

CHAPTER 6

Coping Churn

Metaphorically, coping churn is like a digital loop that keeps playing over and over. A person caught in coping churn has a thought that's stuck; it keeps looping as the mind looks for a resolution. The off switch is not evident and the churning can vary in intensity, duration and frequency. These variables are defined by a person's coping skills. For someone with low coping skills a small event can play loudly and when there's no obvious resolution, the situation is defined as being painful, which to the brain means stop. The options a person chooses to stop pain vary depending on their coping skills.

The root cause of coping churn can vary from little events (e.g., a friend did not return a call) to major events such as divorce. Regardless of the antecedent, the reality is a single event started the loop. The event that triggers coping churn can be compounded when it is repeated over and over, like Sam going to work every day. He's reminded of his stress not only by his thinking but also by his daily interactions with his world. How long a person stays in coping churn defines the degree of risk for experiencing mental illness or other chronic diseases.

The Your Life at Work research through *The Globe and Mail* showed that the coping crisis is a real problem in our society today. Based on the data collected, it's evident that there are many Sams who are not sure how to cope with their current life situation. They characteristically think that they are alone and different than others, as though something is uniquely wrong with them. This can be dangerous because it can inhibit a person from asking for help. Without any situational change, staying in coping churn for an extended period of time can cause a person to lose hope. When this happens, life loses meaning.

Understanding how coping churn works can help to explain why Sam is struggling with his life and engaging in unhealthy behaviours. Like most healthy human beings, Sam is wired to avoid pain and to seek pleasure. But picking pleasure to escape a perceived pain, if the behaviour is unhealthy, can paradoxically result in more pain (e.g., addictive disorders) over the long term. Sam's chronic nights of eating junk food are his weakness; he uses food as his feel-good strategy.

Sam knows that this nightly eating has resulted in his extra body weight. It also explains why he feels more sluggish and is more fatigued. Things that used to be easy are hard. Walking up a set of stairs for him is like climbing a mountain. It's common for him to start to sweat within two minutes of any physical activity. This has become his new norm. As a result, he looks for ways to avoid such activities.

Coping churn happens outside a person's awareness. It's the result of internal conflict that creates pain, which is something to be avoided or stopped. Sam's coping churn is the loop he runs about his work and being sentenced to be alone for the rest of his life. This story runs nonstop. It creates pain daily for Sam. He simply never gets away from his coping churn. This has

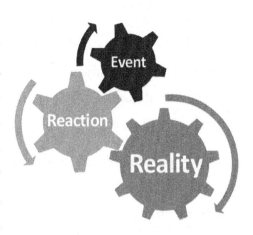

resulted in a build-up of stress, frustration, regret and unresolved conflict. Sam feels like he's failing in life and he's watching a bad movie, which is his life passing him by. To stop coping churn it's worthwhile to understand how it starts.

Event — Coping churn begins with an event. There are two types of events. First come the interactions one has with their environment, such as peer pressure, work demand, manager-employee relationship, bullies/harassment, pay, job, teams and conflict. The second type comes from a person's automatic thoughts, which are the thoughts they create and the value they attach to them with respect to their current life and/or self. Whether the event is externally or internally driven, both do the same thing: they provide a person with information about the event, called a stimulus. Human beings have no choice but to react to stimuli. How one reacts influences their cognitive reality.

Reaction — Once a stimulus is received the person must react. Some believe how they respond is a forced reaction (e.g., he hit me so I had no choice; I hit him back). We have all heard this line of thinking before. It presents the assumption that the person had no choice; they were only reacting to a stimulus. Why? When a person is stuck in coping churn they look to blame the environment as well as to rationalize their behaviour. The danger with this line of thinking is the person may actually come to believe they have no choice.

Many people are simply not aware that every action they take — good or bad — is their choice. Like Sam, who believes he has no choice and his manager's actions are creating his reality at work. Neuroscience and cognitive behavioural science would suggest that each person creates their own mental map, which defines and creates their reality as to what they believe is possible and true.

As mentioned earlier, human beings are motivated to move away from pain and toward pleasure. A key insight for a person to learn how to stop coping churn is to get to the point where they actually believe their thinking is creating their own reality, not what is happening in their environment.

Yes, the environment can encourage and discourage, but it can't control our choices. Granted, sometimes it may feel that way and the option of not conforming to an expected outcome can be severe and unappealing — but you still have a choice.

One element that can exacerbate this reaction is interaction. Interaction refers to how other people react to our reaction, which can be positive or negative. People's reactions can influence coping churn as it often happens outside a person's level of awareness.

Most dog lovers enjoy tossing a ball to their pet. The anticipated reaction when the ball is thrown is that the dog will fetch. When the ball is thrown and the dog doesn't do what is expected, this can influence the owner to work harder to encourage the dog to fetch. Perhaps the dog is tired or just doesn't feel like playing. Some dog owners cope better than others with their dog's reaction.

This simple explanation can help teach the importance of interaction. It provides a frame of reference as to why humans in coping churn can feel worse when their interaction with others is opposite of what they expect. This reaction, if not managed, can have a negative impact on one's coping churn.

As simple as it is, a stimulus is nothing more than information. Others' expectations and belief systems can, if left unchecked, influence one's reaction. The reaction stage is the gap where a person decides what they are going to do or not do. How they react defines their reality. A lot of things can happen in the mind quickly. The person takes an inventory and judges what is happening to them and the risks involved. How they react is influenced by their experiences, beliefs, core competencies and self-confidence in order to cope with the stimulus.

When Sam faces a stimulus that he finds overwhelming, such as coping with his manager, powerful emotions like fear take over. He gets into his getaway-from-pain programming: avoidance. He then uses learned behaviours to attempt to feel better, like eating at night. He's paying a big price that has long-term consequences for short-term relief.

Sam knows eating junk food at night is not good for him but he sees no available alternatives. He has developed this habit as a way to perceive that he's getting relief from pain. Sam without knowing it is caught in what is called a positive feedback loop. The name and the action of positive feedback wording may not sound logical.

The way in which this works is: *(A) stressors leads to (B) learned behaviour, which leads to (A) stressors,* and back to *B (learned behaviour)* and Sam finds himself in a vicious cycle. As a result, Sam thinks about work (stressors) and inevitably tension builds up. His relief is B (his food habit). This leads to feelings of guilt and shame for eating, which results in feeling bad. He continues to eat and the loop continues. A feeds B; B feeds A. Positive feedback loops end with disequilibrium. The system runs in this dysfunctional pattern as long as it can until it breaks. Sam's body is breaking down. If he doesn't change his disequilibrium he will be more at risk for chronic disease or even death.

The solution for Sam is to move from a positive feedback loop to a negative one. Again, the name is not intuitive. Think about a thermostat on a wall. Once the temperature is set at 20 degrees Celsius, when the temperature goes to 21 the furnace turns off; when the temperature drops to 19 the furnace turns on. What is happening is constant feedback and self-correction.

One key coping skill is self-monitoring. People who, for example, use a daily journal to achieve and monitor their life goals often are more successful because they are reflecting, adjusting and correcting on a daily basis. However, to make any change one must be motivated and see the value in making the change. For Sam to take control of his life he will need to break out of the positive feedback loop he has gotten himself stuck in.

Sam often criticizes himself for not being able to figure out how to cope in a healthier manner. Awareness and motivation alone will not create the change needed to be able to react better. For Sam to improve how he reacts he must learn and see that there are alternatives to what he's doing. He also has to believe he can learn and do things differently. How a person reacts defines their reality.

Reality — On the surface, it may sound simple that the life choices Sam makes define his reality. This is where it becomes complicated for people like him. It's programmed into human nature that when someone experiences or perceives pain, the impulse is to get away from it and to look for a way to feel better. The reality for Sam is his reaction often ends up having no impact at addressing the stimulus. His reactions often are shortcuts to create symptom relief to escape from pain. But, as we have seen, his coping skills do not support his physical and mental health.

For example, Sam often goes home at the end of the day frustrated and upset about work. His cure is to sit alone for hours in front of a TV, eating unhealthy junk food. He uses food for symptom relief but every night he feels terrible after all the eating. Each day this memory of feeling bad is removed, but a powerful urge hits him each night to sit down and eat as a way to escape his coping churn. He has constructed a reality where he feels powerless. His tension doesn't ease until he begins eating. Sam may have a food addiction, which is psychologically driven. He's trapped in coping churn.

Coping Churn Impact

Without action and insight into the benefits of developing more effective coping skills in order to change his view of the world, it is unlikely that Sam will do anything differently, and his coping churn may never get resolved. Many people like Sam end up in a coping crisis because they are locked up in coping churn. Without developing new coping skills they stay in coping churn for years — or perhaps for life.

Sam has no family history or genetic predisposition to clinical depression. From a young teen he never quite fit in and struggled to cope with life challenges such as dealing with people. The long-term grind of not being able to cope and being in coping churn for many years has taken a toll.

Sam's coping churn is that he feels "powerless and trapped in this job and life." This loop of self-doubt plays daily for Sam, and with it come powerful emotions: likely hopelessness and depression. Sam is at the point where he believes he has no alternatives with respect to what he can do. He also lives with this secret alone. He doesn't talk to anyone about how he feels or what he thinks. He keeps repeating each day, anticipating it will be the same as the day before.

At this point in his life Sam has not yet put together all the pieces as to how his choices and thinking are facilitating his coping churn. But to be fair to Sam, he's like many people, where the old adage is so true: people simply don't know what they don't know. Sam sees no pathway to coping. His thinking has not evolved to the point where he believes things could ever get better.

Coping churn can be multiplex, meaning a person can be dealing with several different stimuli that are fuelling coping churn. It's not uncommon for there to be a combination of externally and internally driven stimuli. Sam doubts himself daily about how he's coping with his life. His automatic thoughts jump around from various topics (e.g., I'm a failure; I don't like this job; it will never get better; I'm trapped). These thoughts are distracting and painful, and happen all the time. Sam feels trapped in his head and sees no off switch. His think-ing is distracting and comes without warning throughout the day.

In active coping churn, the mind can easily become distracted. Sam, as you recall, was distracted at the set of traffic lights. His mind ran off on him and he lost track of his current reality. He was creating another reality that was elsewhere. His mind was wandering off looking for answers or hiding. Coping churn, when chronic, replays unresolved feelings. One way to start to understand what one can do to stop or reduce coping churn is to start to gain insight

> Do you see how coping churn can lead to developing a mental health issue or several chronic diseases?

on how the mind works. The mind creates the reality that a person believes and lives, whether it's true or not.

Coping Gears

How people behave in coping churn is similar to the five gears in most cars. Their behaviour determines what gear they are in. Each gear represents a mental state.

Park — In this gear the mind wanders and jumps around with no real purpose. Some call this daydreaming. The mind is looking to relax and not work hard; it's easily distracted. A person can go into park through watching TV or surfing the Internet. This mental state allows the mind to become distracted and hide from the challenges of life. When the mind is parked it's not engaged in problem solving or feeling the effects of coping churn. It's busy engaging the world it has created. This mental distraction can be helpful as it sometimes can release tension and pressure that allows the mind to naturally arrive at solutions that can be used to stop or reduce coping churn. However, too much of anything can become a problem. Sam spends hours each day in front of a TV. Little productivity or life change happens due to this unproductive investment of time.

Reverse — In this gear the mind keeps replaying past events. When these are negative they can facilitate a cycle of stress because the person keeps looping and replaying their past events. Each time the brain replays a negative event it can shape a person's perception of themselves. This gear fuels coping churn and the powerful emotions associated with negative experiences. People who replay negative past events also experience them over and over. When a person replays these events the body can become tense as though it were reliving the bad experience.

If there are no alternatives or solutions that meet the person's needs it's typical for them to look for pleasurable ways to distract the mind, though the behaviour that's selected can be self-destructive. The mind often accepts the notion of the behaviour because it has learned that there is some perceived benefit. For example, alcohol can distract the mind to stop thinking about the past, as it numbs the brain. It may feel like a short-term solution but since alcohol is a depressant it rarely helps over the long term and comes with its own host of risks and health problems.

Drive I — In this gear the mind is trying to push through the coping churn. The person knows there's a problem, wants a solution, starts to form ideas and solutions, and sees the value of taking action. They put forth a mental push to get up the courage to take action. All the risks associated with action are top of mind. With these comes emotion and in some cases intense fear and/or anxiety. To move to the next gear the person needs to calm their emotions and feel confident that they can handle the consequences of their action. It's all too common for a person with low coping skills to get stuck at this stage. Too often they fail to muster the courage to take action and as a result give up on their thinking. They then relapse to their learned coping habit that may be negative. Some people create positive habits, such as exercise, to cope. But exercising all the time and not dealing with life can become a problem as well. The negative impact of giving up is that the person perceives they have failed, which often adds to coping churn. The good news about the mind is that automatic thoughts can be both positive and negative. As fast as a person is convinced that they are a failure, the mind can put up a new idea such as making another concerted effort and it is now time to try again. People in this gear may get stuck, like Sam.

It's useful to self-evaluate in which gear you spend your typical day.

Others will spin their wheels for a bit and eventually break out to the next gear and take a chance.

Drive II — In this gear the mind starts to believe it has choices and the potential to take control of the situation. The person now has confidence that they can take action and accept the consequences. They start to process and accept that the only things they have full control over are their actions, and they begin to gain control of their emotions. A key element for evolving coping skills is awareness of who is in control. What people think defines what they do. Sam has not yet found this gear; he hasn't even seen he's in control of his own actions. Moving from the above two gears to this gear often feels like a big weight has been taken off a person's back. This is the gear that stops coping churn. It's common for a person to appear that they are in this gear and making good progress but without notice, relapse to one of the earlier two gears. At this point they slip back into their coping churn. Failing is expected and is normal. Most everyone has heard the example that when learning to ride a bike failure is a part of learning. The issue is not failure. The issue is how after one fails, it takes courage to get back on track and try again. Regardless of how strong a person's coping skills are, life has potholes and seldom is there a perfectly smooth ride. Keeping this in mind can help normalize the fact that humans are not perfect. As well, we are the final judge of our value and worth.

Drive III — In this gear the mind is confident in its ability to cope with life and its challenges. There is no active coping churn. To get to this gear one must understand how developed and matured their coping skills are. The more advanced one's coping skills, the less likely they will be in coping churn, and if they do go into it they will be in it for a shorter period of time. When a person is at this level it does not suggest they may not have slipups. Reaching this gear suggests a person has more traction and capabilities to cope with life and to get back on track when they take a short detour. In this gear they feel confident and in control of their decisions and life; they accept accountability for their thinking and choices. This is a gear that Sam has yet to find for much of his life. He has one exception: when it comes to his work he knows he's skilled and can do it well. He never questions his work ability, just his value. Perhaps that's why he stays in the same job and doesn't look for something that may be better for him.

Coping churn can be short- or long-term. It's common for any person who is hit by a life challenge to experience a setback and spend time in coping churn as they process and take action to cope. The longer a person spends in coping churn, the less likely they will believe, like Sam, that there are any alternatives or hope.

The first step to break out of coping churn is to take responsibility for one's thinking and actions. Not until that happens will a person be ready and motivated to stop coping churn. It's OK to not have the answers or know how to fix one's situation. The journey for better control of one's life is to accept the fact that we own all of our decisions and actions.

To stop coping churn a person needs to find their drive gear. The next chapter reviews the things to consider for one to learn how to slow coping churn, with the ultimate goal to stop coping churn altogether.

CHAPTER 7

Slowing Coping Churn

The demands of work and his manager continue to be the number one source of stress that fuels Sam's coping churn. He knows his manager is demanding but that he most likely would never attack or physically hurt him.

People have tried to influence Sam with little success thus far. For example, he has dismissed his doctor's coaching that his health is slipping because of his lifestyle choices. When Sam is put on depression medication he assumes it is because of all the work stress and to help him cope so he can continue to work. On a daily basis he presents himself to the world with a flat affect; he does not show emotions, good or bad; he keeps things neutral.

Fortunately, Sam has determined that his reality is created by what he thinks, not by what others think. The human brain calibrates and adapts its emotions and drives behaviours based on internal beliefs. These beliefs are not as locked down as much as a person like Sam would like others to believe. With the right situation and influence a person can change their beliefs in short order.

Consider a child playing at home alone who is upset because they can't get what they want. They complain and make a fuss that they won't play until their parents can get them their six red cars. Five is not good enough; they have it in their head that they need all six cars. They cry and complain until the parents tear the house apart and find the sixth car. This creates calm; the child is now able to play happily. After about 15 minutes of playing alone, one of the child's friends shows up to play with them. The child immediately stops playing, confirms the friend wants to play cars, and then happily gives them three of the six cars to play with.

Observers would note that the two children are focused on their cars and not on each other. They both play along, each enjoying their three cars. Clearly, the child who wanted six cars adjusted their belief system for what they needed to be able to play. Their brain perceived and knew that the child now only had three cars and was able to hold back the emotions and enjoy the moment. How is this possible? The brain has an amazing ability to adapt quickly and change its belief system.

What if Sam focused on his IT skills and his proven track record as an IT problem solver? He has lots of good in his life, but because he is hyper-focused on what is not working he has thus far surrendered and allowed his environment to influence his beliefs, thinking and actions. At this point, if something big happened in Sam's environment, such as someone taking a real interest in him and gaining his trust, what would happen to his belief system about being alone? If Sam trusted what was happening was real and embraced it, one healthy, strong relationship could have a major impact and influence on him. There are a multitude of Sams out there whose lives could be improved so much if they were able to have one healthy relationship that could help them by challenging their belief systems.

Life happiness is arguably a balance of skills and luck. Yes, we all need to own our behaviour, but it's important to be pragmatic and practical at the same time. With a bit of luck, Sam may run into that one person with whom he has a connection and build a powerful rapport. A new person in Sam's life could add a new level of thinking. The point here is that every healthy and sane person will cope better with life with a healthy support system, which challenges their belief system and provides healthy alternatives.

Sam has not had luck on his side. He can't create his own luck, though most adults have an experience where they meet one really compatible person because they were at a certain place at a certain time. One problem for people like Sam is when they get stuck in coping churn they believe the only way their life can be improved is when their environment changes. A little luck never hurt anyone, but it's hard to count on and as a result it's a more prudent course to create one's own pathway.

Once a person accepts that they own their behaviours, the next step is to begin to understand how their decisions and choices have shaped their belief system. What we believe shapes our expectations, wants, needs and values. One daily challenge for most of us is how to best manage our expectations, which create our internal rules for what we believe we need in order to be happy. Many have much of what they want in life but can't enjoy it because they are too focused on what they don't yet have. As a result, they forget to acknowledge or celebrate who they are and what they have accomplished in life.

Coping skills operate in the conscious brain. They are dependent on a conscious effort to solve personal and interpersonal problems.[20] They assist a person to navigate powerful emotions that can arise from interaction with the environment, and they are the key to breaking out of coping churn. Whenever a person observes a difference between what they want and what they have they must make a choice and take action. Not making a decision or a choice is still an action.[21]

Sam's coping pathway will define his opportunity for breaking out of coping churn, which will mean taking accountability for his actions, whether good or bad. All anyone can do is take control of their choices; they can't make others do what they don't want to do. Hoping for someone to change in some situation may be in one's self-interest or a conscientious gesture, but ultimately the other person owns their behaviour, too.

Each person's expectations define their reality. Expectations are beliefs that are dynamic and are not always locked in; they can be influenced and changed. Many people simply don't understand that they are constantly redefining their reality through their interpretation of what they have now compared to what they expect. Sam has yet to consider that his perception of his reality is shaded by his focus on what is not working in his life. He theoretically is one conversation away from thinking about his world differently. Beliefs are not as locked down as some may think.

Sam did not always think he would be alone. He had dreams of one day getting married and having love and happiness in his life. As his life unfolded and his unhealthy coping strategy evolved, however, it resulted in isolating himself from people and his dream faded. As a result, Sam has accepted with a sad heart that he will be alone. This story has influenced his belief system.

So if it's true that Sam never planned or wanted to be alone, why doesn't he do something now? It's simple. But simple doesn't mean it's easy to understand or process. Sam has formed an internal belief system that positions the story that his life will be difficult, that he will be alone each and every day. It's Sam's Groundhog Day; he expects to live each day the same way. Keeping his expectations low is Sam's strategy to protect himself from risk of failure and pain. All the pain associated with his life choices is just a tax he's paying to obtain the outcome he so much wants: peace.

Sam is not alone in not taking risks. To get out of coping churn requires a decision and sometimes taking a chance. Think about the guy in a bar. As he looks over and sees what he perceives as an interesting and beautiful woman, he says to himself, *"Wow!"* But the thought of going over to introduce himself is overwhelming.

It's safer for him to feel alone versus making it official by introducing himself. Why? The belief is in his head that the woman will reject him, so to avoid rejection he doesn't take a chance. Onlookers who observe Sam may not understand the fear of failure that holds him and many others back. The perceived pain of failure keeps them in their current reality and belief.

One tragic reality is that in coping churn there is never truly any peace; only pain and consequences. Sam has formed the belief that his evening routine gives him peace. But this is just an illusion that creates a minor escape from his coping churn. He's not happy and he knows it. But like the man at the bar he's safe in his quiet failure. Human logic is not always rational; Sam's thinking is influenced by his cognitive dissonance.

Cognitive dissonance can be defined as a mental stress that is a result of a person holding two contradictory beliefs at the same time. Sam wants to have no conflict with the external world. He has created the internal rule for himself that it's best for him to be alone. Though this is painful, for Sam it's the lesser of two evils. He has aligned his daily cognitions and actions that have resulted in rationalizing that he will always be alone and that is in his best interest. He believes he is living out the cards that he was dealt.

Coping in Action

The first step for slowing down Sam's coping churn is to gain insight into how he responds to a situation that defines how he will cope. Figure 7-1 provides a visual overview of *Coping in Action*. This diagram flows from left to right, showing a breakdown of the coping process. It's meant to show the different drivers and decisions that result in healthy or unhealthy behaviours. Sam, as you will see, has hardwired a pattern as to how he copes with his manager. Breaking a coping crisis starts with learning how one thinks and how their thinking influences their behaviour. Ultimately, it will be in Sam's best interest to unlearn ineffective coping churn and to create new thinking that will be able to better manage stimuli.

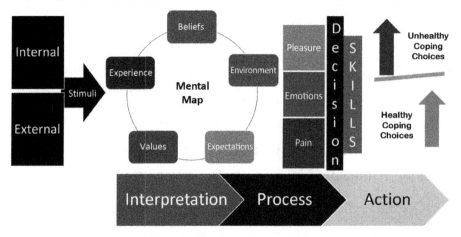

Figure 7-1 — Coping in Action

Interpretation:

Stimuli — As earlier discussed in coping churn, stimuli can be external and internal, and once they are received a person has no choice but to behave (i.e., take action or do nothing, which is also an action).

The Mental Map — This is how the brain starts to break down the meaning of the stimuli. Each person's mental map is their reality of what they expect, believe and can do to manage their life. The mental map influences the kinds of decisions a person generates. Following is an overview of the different elements that influence and shape one's mental map:

- **Experiences** — Education, parenting, mentors, personal and professional involvements. Experience becomes a person's onboard expertise that evolves over their lifetime. Experience provides an opportunity for learning that can shape a person's mental map. Through experience, a person has an opportunity to develop the skills that will influence how effectively they react to stimuli. This is much different than book smarts; it's life smarts that one develops, and these are always evolving.

- **Beliefs** — These are the rules and preferences a person forms and agrees to about themselves and others. The challenge is that they are not always rational — some can be irrational. Sam has formed the belief that he will be alone for his entire life. He has created this from his interactions from being a single child, school experiences, parenting, social interaction, and so forth that have shaped his beliefs with respect to the benefits of being alone — even though it continues to take a toll on him. With 7 billion people on the planet, it's irrational for Sam to think there is no one for him and that he has to be alone. His irrational belief is forming his reality. Beliefs can be positive or negative. They are created by the person. Some are formed automatically without any debate; they are taken on like law. Beliefs influence what a person believes is possible.

- **Environment** — This includes a person's support systems and resources, such as relationships, financial stability, and access to professional resources, which include employee and family assistance, doctors and accountants. It's what the person knows they have access to in their environment that can support or guide them in time of need. Being pack animals, it's healthy for humans to look outside themselves for support. The environment can provide both positive and negative elements. Ultimately, one's mental map will shape how one copes and interacts with their environment.

- **Values** — Different than beliefs, values attach emotions to what is good or bad or neutral. It's how humans code the world emotionally; how they prioritize their life. For example, Sam has put his career in the number one spot. He has yet to value his health. Values influence human decisions. When an employee doesn't agree or support their employer's values this can be a point of contention.

- **Expectations** — This is what the person expects and wants to happen. Every person may have different expectations. This defines what will meet their needs for money, work, relationships, self and health. Values influence how a person sets their expectations. Expectations can be micro-detailed, e.g., how one expects a person to talk to them, reply to them, the time it takes for them to reply, and the medium they use to reply.

The mental map influences the emotions associated with and interpretation of a stimulus as being pain or pleasure. Again, human beings have no choice but to act. Action requires a decision based on one's skills and experiences. The decisions and skills collectively influence the way a person handles the stimulus with respect to their coping choice. Coping in action provides a framework that demonstrates how a person's decisions drive coping churn. The brain works fast. It's able to quickly attach a value to information (stimulus). When the brain receives the stimulus it's labelled as positive, neutral or negative.

The degree of Sam's mental map maturity defines his ability to cope. Coping skills are trainable and they evolve as one starts to become aware of how each piece of their mental map shapes and influences their decisions and actions. Developing coping skills improves a person's confidence and competency to cope with the vagaries of life.

Coping Continuum

How a person regularly copes with stimuli defines where they fall in Figure 7-2 — Coping Continuum, which shows the outcome of one's coping skills. The manner in which a person copes can be put into five categories. This continuum is aligned with the mental health continuum. It's not by chance that a person's coping skill choices can predict their current and future mental health.

- *At-Risk coping* — The purpose of at-risk coping is to move away from pain. The person who is determined to or takes a chance engaging in at-risk behaviour, in the moment, brings more opportunities for pleasure and distracting pain. Engaging in unhealthy habits to feel better is often done with little evaluation of short- and long-term risk. The focus is on the now. The person wants to move away from pain. Factors often associated with at-risk coping include alcohol, drugs, gaming, Internet, shopping, sexting, pornography and food, all of which make a high percentage of people feel good in the moment. They all create the illusion of control over a situation. The downside is they don't effectively access the root cause or solve underlying problems; they only remove or dissociate the individual

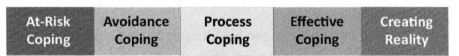

Figure 7-2 — Coping Continuum

from them. The problems are typically waiting for them once they come back from their distracting behaviours.

- *Avoidance coping* — Can be a variety of behaviours, such as making no choices (which is a choice), or avoiding anxiety provoking people, places and things as a strategy to cope. The motivation is the person does not believe they have the resources or skills to address the challenging situation they face or that is challenging them. Many don't like conflict so they are motivated internally to avoid it, as they associate conflict with pain. Avoiding something clearly doesn't solve the issue. Cognitive dissonance can come into play here. One example is how Sam has talked himself into a story as to why it's OK to be alone.

- *Process coping* — Refers to the process a person goes through to cope. Some people become upset and show lots of emotion before they calm down, apologize and move on. The person typically goes through some process and that takes a toll on them. They have to use energy to get through emotions. They may also need time to get through their emotions. Time can vary from a few hours to days to even weeks and months. Once the person is able to get their emotions under control they are in a position to start to process the situation and look at their options to cope. In this stage they can begin engaging in healthy behaviours as a way to cope that helps them become stable. Much like coming out of a fog, they are able to see their situation with a clear lens, make healthier decisions, and cope more effectively.

- *Effective coping* — This is healthy coping where the person is able to react to what's in front of them in a healthy and safe manner to themselves and others. They are still reacting, however, to the environment more than leading it. This is OK. It's just important to point out that the person is waiting for life to happen more than creating it. This is the level a person needs to be at to avoid coping churn.

- *Creating reality* — This is the ultimate coping style. This is an entirely different mindset. The person is not focusing on coping with life but creating it. They are able to deal with the setbacks and challenges they face. They are driven from within to lead themselves to confidently create their own reality. These people are leaders and innovators. They make things happen instead of waiting for them to happen.

Healthy coping choices build a person's confidence in themselves and thus their competency; they help promote and create calm and peace. Developing one's coping skills can be hard work. The goal is to reduce risk for coping churn, thus creating one's own reality rather than simply reacting to it.

Whatever category of coping in which a person spends the majority of time influences their sense of hope. Hope is the belief there could be something better.

Sam has made many choices that have put his health at risk. He has always, however, made the choice to live. Consequently, he may not see a path for changing his life. However, he still found some light of hope at the moment he questioned whether to live or die. What if Sam allowed himself an opportunity to learn or explore options to improve his life? It could be a major insight and learning opportunity for Sam to realize how the coping-in-action framework provides insight that his approach to coping puts him at risk of ending up on the wrong end of the coping continuum.

Improving coping skills does not require a lot of decisions; it requires only accepting responsibility for one's decisions. This, in essence, is taking accountability for one's life and actions. The next action is to be open to learn how to develop coping skills. This can be accomplished by seeking an answer to the question: "How can I develop my coping skills?" A useful support system to engage with might include your doctor, employee and family assistance counsellor, psychologist, social worker, professional therapist, local university, community resources or the Internet. Asking this question is a good step. The next is following up and making a concerted effort to take action.

It's evident that people can develop healthier coping skills. The evidence is in front of us: millions of people in North America go to professional counsellors, therapists or psychiatrists each week looking for answers for how to better cope. Many get relief and solutions. Many do not due to the fact that they have not developed effective coping skills. In other words, they failed to learn to cope.

Those who make an effort to learn coping skills are making a decision that in time will improve their quality of life. One fortunate fact is coping skills can be taught and help people like Sam. There might be fewer Sams if coping skills were developed earlier in one's life. This activity would reduce individuals' risk for developing psychosocial-driven mental health issues. The coping crisis can be averted with early intervention or, better yet, prevention.

Many adults have never been trained or learned how to develop their coping skills, which influence personal decision making. There is no surprise that today we are in a coping crisis. The facts are clear. Many people like Sam knowingly make poor decisions daily in an effort to cope with stress. The way to curb a coping crisis is early intervention: for people to learn coping skills at an early age. Whether a person wants to learn to ride a bike, read or write, or cope better they need to do the work required. Society can't do the work for them.

To impact the current coping crisis will require effort from individuals; the crisis can't be solved by a societal mandate. It will only be curbed one person at a time. Each person's mental health and happiness are dependent on how well they learn to cope with life.

The first rule is to keep an untroubled spirit. The second is to look things in the face and know them for what they are.
If you are pained by external things, it is not they that disturb you, but your own judgement of them. And it is in your power to wipe out that judgment now.
Think of what you have rather than of what you lack. Of the things you have, select the best and then reflect how eagerly you would have sought them if you did not have them. — Marcus Aurelius

CHAPTER 8

Road Map to Better Coping

Developing one's coping skills begins with learning and understanding how the mind works; it's analogous to learning how to ski, which requires motivation, conscious choice, persistence, and dedication. It takes practice and the expectation that prior to the mastery of coping skills there will be failure. Good intentions are not sufficient for success. Developing a habit requires learning from failure and moving a skill from being a conscious effort, to effortless; making the mastery of coping skills a natural part of life.

Individuals who learn and understand coping in action and the coping continuum are in a position to start to take accountability for how they successfully manage their decisions and actions. This will help to shine a light on a healthier, more effective coping pathway.

Luckily, Sam has decided to go to counselling. The breakthrough was accepting that it was his choices that created his current reality. His counsellor helped soften this reality by suggesting to Sam that people can only do what they know and believe.

Sam is intrigued that through talk therapy these conversations are starting to influence his belief system and he is beginning to realize that this counselling could have a positive, cascading effect on his life. Once he learned about coping churn he found it interesting with respect to how he talked himself into being alone. More importantly, though it was not what he truly wanted, somehow he convinced himself that it was tolerable. His IT work-oriented brain was able to process the coping in action model and saw how his mental map was shaping his choices to escape pain.

Sam has had a breakthrough; he now accepts responsibility for his actions. Not knowing what to do, he went to see his family doctor to make a plan. He was ready to take responsibility for his actions, but didn't know how to change for the better. His doctor was pleased to hear Sam decide to change his story and to break the coping crisis he has been in for years. Sam also made an appointment with a counsellor referred to him by his doctor. His goal was to change his story. He was a bit nervous and wondered if talking about it could actually make things worse.

Sam made a proactive decision by going to counselling to seek guidance on how to develop the core competency he needs to improve his coping skills. He has accepted that his choices have been negatively impacting his quality of life and he's starting to understand that much of his coping crisis is due to a lack of awareness with respect to how he has been coping with stress. He also knows that developing his coping skills starts with accepting that he's accountable for his choices — all of them — whether they are good or bad.

Sam is excited to get to the point where he can start to successfully manage the powerful emotions of fear that for years have driven old habits and poor choices. With his counsellor he now has a clear understanding of the five life tasks he has been struggling with and how stress attacks both the mind and body. He also appreciates the interplay between the conscious and unconscious mind, and the power of emotions that drive behaviours such as fear. He has also gained valuable insight on the concepts of coping churn and coping in action. He knows why he ended up where he was on the coping continuum, as well as the relationship between this continuum and mental illness.

Sam now has insight on the coping pathway with respect to how coping is mastered. He now needs to explore the different kinds of core competencies that will help him improve his ability. His counsellor has suggested that he take coping skills training in addition to counselling.

One option is a nine-week program called *Pathway to Coping,* offered through the University of New Brunswick, which is 100 percent on-demand, online learning (see Appendix A). The purpose of these kinds of programs is to provide people like Sam an opportunity to explore in depth key building blocks for developing coping skills.

In counselling, Sam was provided an introduction to several key pieces that are important to help a person start to develop their coping skills. Sam's counsellor used the following three-step framework called *1-2-3 I Can Cope* to guide Sam on his journey to develop his coping skills.

1-2-3 I Can Cope

Step 1 Awareness — The first step was for Sam to develop a baseline of his current coping capabilities. It was recommended that Sam pursue the free Your Life at Work resource[23] published in *The Globe and Mail*. The resource includes three survey tools that help a person determine a baseline of how they are coping with life stress (see Appendix B for links to surveys):

- *Quality of Work Life* (for employees in a workplace who are interested in evaluating how their coping skills affect their overall health)

- *Quality of Life* (for individuals looking to evaluate how they are coping with their life overall)

- *Quality of Student Life* (for high school, college and university students looking for insight on how well they are coping with the demands of school)

Each of these three tools is designed to provide a benchmark outlining the manner in which a person is coping with stress and how that relates to their engagement and health. Our research through *The Globe and Mail* has found that coping skills are a lead indicator. This research supports the findings from my doctoral research that revealed coping skills are a moderator (i.e., evidence of the role coping skills play) between perceived stress and health, meaning people with more advanced coping skills on average have a lower health risk and are better able to engage in life in a proactive and healthy manner.

Sam chose the *Quality of Life* tool. He took his time and read the articles on Jack and Jill (see Appendix B), which helped him

Figure 8-1
Indicate the percentage of time your mind spends in each category each day.
Note: The percentages cannot total more than 100%.

Past	NOW	Future

start to realize that he was not alone and to see the role and impact that coping skills can have on a person's quality of life.

Sam's counsellor asked him where his mind spends the majority of its time with respect to past, present, and future (see Figure 8-1). His counsellor helped Sam see the value of developing his coping skills. It required Sam's focus on the NOW.

The counsellor wanted Sam to know that the mind, when it is left unsupervised, often will jump around from the past to the future. This focus on past and potential future failures leads to unnecessary grief and anxiety, particularly if the past situation is linked to coping churn. The counsellor felt it was important to make the point to Sam that automatic thoughts often come without notice.

Sam was asked to think about where his mind goes when he feels his manager has been rude to him. The counsellor wanted Sam to understand that it is quite normal to have random thoughts. It's not the thoughts that matter as much as what one does with them. The counsellor wanted Sam to gain insight on the point that it's quite normal for the unconscious mind to create some interesting ideas that the conscious mind quickly shuts down or accepts.

His counsellor helped Sam realize that some of his choices were created by the unconscious mind. He found it particularly important to make the point that when the conscious mind does not shut down, automatic thoughts can start to influence emotions, thoughts and behaviours, which can initiate coping churn. Sam started to see how he had more than one story involving coping churn that impacted how he was behaving both at home and at work. To help normalize the concept of coping churn the counsellor helped Sam understand that the human mind is quite capable of having multiple stories running at once.

Sam learned the average person typically spends less than 20 percent of their mental energy focusing on the now. It's not uncommon for people to replay yesterday's news over and over as if it were an extension of now. If the story is painful it most likely is coping churn. This was referred to earlier as the reverse gear.

Sam is fascinated by how his mental map is based on what he thinks about his current reality. His internal conversations have been his reality. Sam has accepted that his reality is created inside out and not outside in. He acknowledged to his counsellor that one of his big "ah hah" moments was that his coping skills ultimately determine how any stimuli are dealt with.

Sam completed his *Quality of Work Life* benchmark, determined his current coping skills baseline and saw how coping skills were impacting his engagement and health. His counsellor's follow-up session covered the following questions:

Step 1 — Follow-Up

- What did you learn from completing your assessment?
- What percentage of time do you spend in the present moment?
- Are you currently experiencing any coping churn?
- Over the past six months, where do you fall on the coping continuum?
- If you improved your coping skills, how could it have a positive impact on your life? Be specific: what would be improved?

Sam is pleased he has taken this first step. He now has more insight on coping than he ever had. He appreciates how his counsellor is breaking down his coping crisis into easy and digestible matters he can relate to. Sam asked his counsellor why he was not formally taught coping skills in the years he spent in the education system. The counsellor's response: "Sam I'm not sure on the why, I just know the need and value. So perhaps with all the concerns with mental health more organizations, including the education system, will focus more time and energy on teaching coping skills."

Step 2 Inventory — The second step the counsellor took with Sam was to create a detailed inventory of his available environmental support resources that he can tap into to help him cope with life. The counsellor wanted to make the point that we all are accountable for our own choices but that doesn't mean we will not benefit from support systems. Every person will benefit from healthy and supportive relationships. It's healthy to have someone who is trusted to run ideas by, as well as who can call one out on choices that may not be in their best interest. The counsellor wanted Sam to know that no one is perfect; we all are fallible and we all make mistakes. Sam is quickly learning that counselling is working for him as it's helping provide a framework that facilitates accountability. The counsellor told Sam the *Pathway to Coping* program will only help reinforce this concept as the tool includes weekly lessons and activities to use for self-monitoring.

Environmental Factors

Sam completed the activity in Table 8-1 in order to evaluate the support resources he has in place.

Sam's counsellor wanted him to start to grasp the fact that human beings are pack creatures; they do better in a safe and healthy pack than alone. Sam had more liabilities than assets. His counsellor assured him that through developing his coping skills he will be able to move liabilities to assets.

Table 8-1 — Environmental Factors		
Evaluate each item below as an asset or liability; the item cannot be both. Check one option for each and then count your checkmarks to determine your ratio of assets to liabilities. The objective is to find your current benchmark. As you develop your coping skills you can move items from liabilities to assets.	Asset	Liability
1. Family — loving and caring family support		
2. Partner — loving and caring partner		
3. Money — financial stability		
4. Work — in a paid or non-paying role you enjoy and find rewarding		
5. Housing — in safe and clean housing that meets your requirements		
6. Support systems (e.g., employee and family assistance program, community, family doctor) — have access to resources to leverage in the event of need		
Total		

Sam started to imagine how helpful it would be to have a loving, supportive partner and friends who care to talk to him on a daily basis. He also started to see that a part of this process is to help him gain confidence to address his perceived stressors and fears so he can move forward. Sam has all the material pieces of his life in place: job, money and housing. What he's missing is the people piece.

Important Life Values

The next lesson the counsellor wanted to approach with Sam was the importance of prioritization. We make a priority to spend energy on the things that we value the most. The counsellor wanted Sam to understand that the exception to this rule is addictive behaviours. His counsellor helped Sam understand that he had developed a food addiction.

Sam's counsellor had him complete a food addiction screen (see Appendix C) because he used food to feel good as a reward. As much as Sam thought about trying to be disciplined with regard to food, his urges triumphed and he ate his nightly serving of junk food.

The challenge with addiction is that it can be psychological and physical. Chemicals like alcohol and other drugs create powerful physical addictions, thereby reinforcing the addiction by the threat of withdrawal symptoms that occur when one tries to stop feeding the addiction. Once a person feels ill they seek more of the addictive substance in order to feel better.

Psychological addictions like food can be powerful as well. For most addictions there are stress triggers that drive the behaviour. The trigger is a stimulus that encourages the body to find the fastest way to curb the pain. Psychological addictions are powerful as they create the illusion of relief. Sam realized his food addiction was blocking him from valuing his health and self-respect; he was not happy with his body or his current fitness level. His counsellor once again wanted to normalize to Sam that he is not alone. Many people get trapped in habits that are not in their best interest as a way to escape.

Sam's counsellor went on to discuss and support Sam in the development of a plan designed to control his food intake, as well as how to build a relapse prevention program. He told Sam that there's a good chance he will slip but to not focus on the negative. Stumbling blocks are also learning opportunities; "What caused me to slip?" "How can I better deal with that in the future?" It's not the slip the counsellor wants Sam to measure, it's how long it takes him to get back on track after a slip. The counsellor then moved the conversation on to the importance of values.

Sam was introduced to the notion that the degree to which a person values each of the following items will influence their commitment and motivation to take action. In Table 8-2, Sam was asked to evaluate how important each of six important life values was to him today. It was made clear that there are many more things a person can value than are on the list. This list was developed to focus on elements aligned to support a person's success with respect to the five life challenges.

It's not the strongest who survive, nor the most intelligent, but the ones most adaptable to change. — Charles Darwin

Table 8-2 — Important Life Values	
Value	Rating
1. Health (mind and body)	High — Medium — Low — NA
2. Relationship	High — Medium — Low — NA
3. Community	High — Medium — Low — NA
4. Work	High — Medium — Low — NA
5. Money	High — Medium — Low — NA
6. Self (self-esteem)	High — Medium — Low — NA

Being a smart fellow, Sam began to see how his coping skills were playing a role in shaping his current physical and psychological health. It became clear during this exercise that he had not been valuing himself or his health as being important life values to focus on. The counsellor encouraged Sam to see how his environment and values had played a role in his coping pathway. Sam was given an opportunity to change his pathway, but he'll need to do the work; no one can do it for him, and there are no shortcuts.

Sam is now ready to move forward to develop his coping skills. His internal conversations have been his reality. During a session his counsellor asked, "Sam, why are you really here?"

Sam replied, "It's clear to me now. I've decided it's time to cope more effectively with my life. I have not been doing that well and I now know that to take charge I must own my choices. I don't know how long this will take before I feel much better, but I do feel better knowing that there is a pathway and that I am not alone. People who are stuck in situations similar to mine can learn how to live a healthier life that is interesting. I'm just glad the day has come."

Step 2 — Follow-Up

- How confident are you in your environmental support systems?
- Are there any surprises about how you valued health and self?

The counsellor had Sam do the above value exercise. Sam noticed that before this day he most likely never valued himself or his health. After a few sessions with the counsellor Sam started to see how his decisions had shaped his life. He was now ready to change.

Step 3 Motion — Sam has made a decision to make a change and to do so he knows he will need to continue to learn and to take action. He's now in motion. He's in counselling, he's open to learn and, importantly, he takes ideas home to practice.

The counsellor is committed to work with Sam to develop the knowledge and skills that will support his ability to cope with life. As well, Sam has agreed to take a nine-week coping skills training course on his own time. Change starts with awareness, and Sam finally is aware. He has accepted that he's the captain of his own ship. He's not 100 percent sure yet how to steer, but he knows it's his ship to steer.

During Sam's meetings with his counsellor he began a journey to explore key themes that influence one's coping skills. In each session the counsellor took a theme or two and discussed them with Sam. He would then send Sam home after each meeting with homework and items to work on between counselling sessions. The counsellor made it clear that the real work happens outside of counselling, where one starts to practice and take ownership of their skills.

Following is a summary of the themes that Sam explored in counselling:

- **Locus of control** — There are two ends to this continuum. One is called external locus of control. People at this end of the continuum adopt the perspective that the external world determines or is a major influence on their circumstances and choices. Sam could relate strongly to this theme. In the past, when his manager gave him a difficult assignment and short timeframes Sam felt he was powerless. Internal locus of control is the belief that the external world only provides information and each person is accountable for their own choices. Thus, the manager's actions towards Sam may not have been a great experience, but from an internal locus of control perspective, the employee believes they have a choice as to how they will respond. Sam started to understand that going home and feeling sorry for himself was not helping him, especially all the snacking and night eating. Working from an internal locus of control perspective helped Sam remove the emotions of feeling weak for not standing up for himself. He's now learning how to step back and think about his options for resolving his problems in a constructive way (e.g., talk to his manager about timelines and expectations). The internal locus of control position is one that is clearly more advantageous and less influenced by external stressors, though this does not mean an internally focused person does not experience stress. What is important is that this is not a personality trait; it can be developed through awareness and practice.

- **Emotional intelligence (EQ)** — Sam was introduced to the notion that emotional intelligence influences how effectively a person manages to be positive, motivated, empathetic, conscientious and socially competent.[24] EQ helps explain why some people have more capacity for recognizing their own feelings and those of others; for motivating themselves; and for managing emotions in themselves and in their relationships. By learning how to develop his EQ, Sam discovered it helped him to better control his emotions and have more empathy for himself. The greater the person's ability in each area, the higher their emotional intelligence. EQ is a better predictor of an employee's ability to perform in a workplace than IQ. Emotional intelligence can be learned, whereas IQ is often locked in place. Sam knew he was smart in his role and had the IQ to be successful. What he was pleased with was the opportunity to explore how EQ could help him develop more insight on managing and controlling his emotions.

- **Optimistic vs. pessimistic** — Sam learned in counselling that he was basically a pessimistic person. This means Sam typically expects the worst to happen, and he often seeks out the worst.[25] Sam's pessimistic state resulted in experiencing more anxiety, stress and potential health issues on a daily basis, as compared to an optimist. He learned that an optimistic person has the gift of positive reappraisal.[26] This is their ability to see the positive side of a cup that is half full. A person who lives in an optimistic state is better positioned to process life stressors. This is not to suggest that pessimistic people are doomed. Pessimism helps in decision making with respect to being cautious. Sam was pessimistic about his future and as a result when things did not change he was correct in his assessment. He discovered in counselling that he could learn how to become more optimistic and the benefits of looking for the good and the opportunity versus sentencing oneself to failure as a way to manage expectations. Sam realized, *"No wonder I'm depressed, I have always thought I was going to fail in my relationships."*

- **Learning awareness** — The counsellor wanted Sam to know that he is a learning machine, that he is able to learn positive and negative habits. He was taught a concept called vicarious learning (also known as observational learning), which teaches that all human learning can originate from observing another's behaviour.[27] Sam did not have a positive role model. Humans can learn without ever necessarily performing a behaviour or receiving any kind of reward (positive or negative). As a result, people can learn both good and bad habits from observing others. Sam's isolation stopped him from having social interactions where he could learn new skills. The counsellor wanted Sam to think about the kinds of skills he could learn by interacting with people, such as simple social interaction, simple conversation, and how people build strong, healthy relationships through listening, communication and being consistent.

- **Self-efficacy** — Sam was introduced to the concept of how self-efficacy influences his internal beliefs. It defines how confident he is when he wakes up in the morning that he will be able to get through the day effectively.[28] Sam's counsellor explained how developing his self-efficacy will require developing self-competencies (knowledge and skills) such as social interaction, conflict resolution, assertiveness and communication. This will help Sam develop self-esteem. It's plausible to make the assumption that the higher the level of self-efficacy, the higher the probability that Sam will be better able to cope with his work stress. Each person's job defines the kinds of core competency required to form communication, leadership, management and technical skills. A person can have high coping skills but due to other skill gaps they continue to fail in their role. When dealing with the issue of why a person like Sam has stress in their job it's of value to assess whether the cause is a lack of coping skills or gaps in their functional core competency.

Step 3 — Follow-Up

- What actions will you take to expand your knowledge and skills for each of the above five themes (e.g., readings, courses)?

- What is one learning you can take from each of the five themes that you can apply today?

Sam has started the process for developing his coping skills through his counsellor. His desired outcome is to learn how to navigate his coping churn so he can make healthier decisions under pressure. He knows it's time to break old habits and start new ones and he's starting to feel better about owning his life and being accountable for his actions. His counsellor was able to help Sam normalize his situation to realize that he is not atypical. He also helped Sam come to the realization that he is not alone; however, the most important learning is that people in a situation like Sam's have learned how to change their life for the better. Sam is understanding for the first time that there's hope he can have a better life.

Sam has been interested in every meeting with his counsellor. He enjoys his counsellor's insight and encouragement.

Sam is quickly learning that every person will be faced with confronting and coping with both life and work stressors. There is

> *All human actions have one or more of these seven causes: chance, nature, compulsion, habit, reason, passion, and desire.*
> *It is possible to fail in many ways...while to succeed is possible only in one way.*
> *In poverty and other misfortunes of life, true friends are a sure refuge. The young they keep out of mischief; to the old they are an aid and a comfort in their weakness, and those in the prime of life they incite to noble deeds.*
> *You will never do anything in this world without courage. It is the greatest quality of the mind next to honour.*
> *We are what we repeatedly do, excellence then is not an act but a habit.*
> —Aristotle

no escape and it has nothing to do with luck — life happens. Where there are people there will be conflict because we all see the world differently and have different expectations. There's no escaping this fact.

Hiding and avoiding life has been Sam's approach thus far. But in counselling he is learning that stress comes in all shapes and forms. Some stressors are real; some are perceived. It was an important realization for Sam when he learned that stress can be generated from the external world, from one's unconscious mind (automatic) or conscious mind. When not dealt with properly it's common and predictable that the stimuli will drive the stress response. In this state people have no choice but to act. The counsellor reminded Sam of the famous umpire saying what is applicable to all human beings: "It ain't nuthin' till I call it." Meaning when life sends Sam information only Sam can determine if it is constructive or destructive, helpful or unhelpful.

In Figure 8-2, the pathway to health is through coping skills. This visual demonstrates that all life and work stress is processed and dealt with internally. Sam finally has arrived at the point where he knows his future depends on his actions and commitment to learning and practising coping skills. Sam has also learned he may make a bad call here and there, but accepting it and owning these calls is key for him to get back on track. Sam's counsellor helped him realize that setting impossible standards sets a person up for failure.

Sam accepts the notion that learning coping skills is a developmental process, where failure and slipping into old habits is

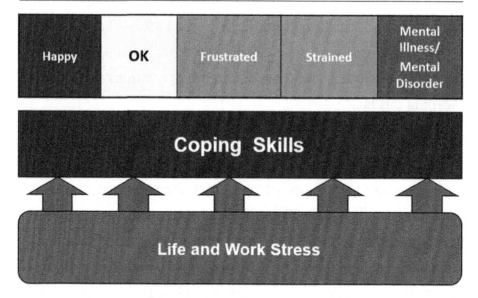

Figure 8-2 — The Pathway to Health

normal. It's not the failure that defines success; it's how long the person who fails takes to try again.

Sam's path to developing his coping skills has begun. He has committed to counselling for the next six months, two times per month, as well as completing the nine-week *Pathway to Coping Skills* training. He understands he has just begun his journey. He has set modest goals, and he and his doctor continue to work together to engage him safely into physical exercise. He's going to focus on diet, hydration and walking for the next three months to build up some endurance, although he doesn't want to open too many fronts.

Each evening now, instead of watching TV he's online working his Pathway to Coping program, doing his assessment, reading and watching YouTube stories that inspire him. It's not a perfect plan, but it's Sam's plan

FOOTNOTES

Chapter 2

1: Lazarus, R. S. (2000). Evolution of a model of stress, coping and discrete emotion. In V. R. Rice (Ed.), *Handbook of stress, coping and health.* Thousand Oaks, CA; Sage.

2: Howatt, W. (2013). Introducing the *Quality of Work Life* Study (QWL) White Paper version 2.4.

3: http://www.theglobeandmail.com/report-on-business/careers/career-advice/life-at-work/

Chapter 3

4: http://www.mentalhealthcommission.ca/English/system/files/private/document/Investing_in_Mental_Health_FINAL_Version_ENG.pdf

5: Canadian Occupational Safety. http://www.cos-mag.com/psychological-safety/psychological-safety-stories/4587-new-study-launched-on-mental-health-in-mining.html

6: http://www.amazon.ca/Talop-Beyond-Engagement-William-Howatt/dp/0992057116

7: http://suicideprevention.ca/understanding/suicide-and-high-risk-groups/

8: Glasser, W. (2000). *Choice theory.* New York. Harper Collins.

9: Petri, H. (1997). *Motivation: Theory, research and applications (4th Ed).* Pacific Grove, CA: Brooks/Cole.

10: Jacobs, C. (2010). *Management rewired.* New York: Penguin Books.

11: https://www.psychologytoday.com/blog/what-doesnt-kill-us/201301/coping-crisis.

12: Selye, H. (1976). *Stress and life.* New York: McGraw-Hill.

13: Glasser, W. (1984). *Control theory.* New York. Harper Collins.

14: Ellis, A. (1980). *Growth through thought.* Palo Alto, CA: Science and

Behaviour Books.

15: Edelwich, J. & Brodsky, A. (1980). *Burnout: Stages of disillusionment in the helping professions.* New York: Human Sciences Press.

16: Lazarus, R. S. (1991). Progress on a cognitive-motivational-relational theory of emotion. *American Psychologist, 46,* 819-834.

17: Lazarus, R. S. (1993). From psychology stress to the emotions: A history of changing outlooks. In L. W. Porter and M. R. Rosenzweig (Eds.). *Annual review of psychology,* 44, 1-21.

18: Lazarus, R. S. (1999). *Stress and emotion.* New York: Springer Publisher.

19: Gershaw, D. A. (1997). Dealing with frustration. Arizona Western College, Psychology Department. Retrieved March 30, 2004, from http://www3.azwestern.edu/psy/dgershaw/lol/frustration2.html.

20: Plotnik (2002). *Introduction to psychology (6ᵗʰ ed).* Pacific Grove, CA: Thomson Learning.

Chapter 7

21: Snyder, C.R. (ed.) (1999) *Coping: The Psychology of What Works.* New York: Oxford University Press.

22: Glasser, W. (2000). *Choice theory.* New York: Harper Collins.

Chapter 8

23: http://www.theglobeandmail.com/report-on-business/careers/career-advice/life-at-work/

24: Goleman, D. (1998). *Emotional intelligence in the workplace.* New York: Bantam.

25: Seligman, M. E. P. (1989). *Helplessness.* New York: Freeman.

26: Seligman, M. E. P. (2002). *Authentic happiness: Using the new positive psychology to realize your potential for lasting fulfillment.* New York: Free Press/Simon and Schuster.

27: Bandura, A. (1986). *Social foundation of thought and action: A social cognition theory.* Englewood Cliffs, NJ: Prentice-Hall.

28: Bandura, A. (1997). *Self-efficacy: The exercise of control.* New York: Freeman.

Appendix C

29: Robert Holman Coombs (Editor) *Handbook of addictive disorders: A practical guide to diagnosis and treatment.* http://ca.wiley.com/WileyCDA/WileyTitle/productCd-0471235024.html
30: http://www.webmd.com/mental-health/mental-health-food-addiction

NOTES

APPENDIX A

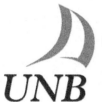

College of Extended Learning

UNB Pathway to Coping Skills

UNIVERSITY OF
NEW BRUNSWICK

By Dr. William Howatt

This program has been designed to be delivered over nine weeks. It is one option to support employees on their pathway to developing coping skills. It makes no claims other than it is committed to providing employees with a structured curriculum for the development of coping skills.

There are two options:

The first option is self-directed — where learner self-paces over nine weeks. They get access to the UNB online learning platform Pathway to Coping course where they will find the curriculum, videos, worksheets and an e-book to support their learning, are provided with the ability to email questions to a coping coach, and to interact in a confidential blog with peers also taking the course to share ideas and encouragement.

The second option includes the same as the above with the addition of a weekly call with a coping coach who will lead in a 90-minute webinar where the coach will review the weekly curriculum and encourage participants to practice their weekly learnings. The logic is that over the nine weeks the learner will be exposed to nine core competencies that have been selected as building blocks to help them get on the right pathway to coping.

The curriculum is presented using a three-stage model that includes a foundational stage of three grounding core competencies for developing coping skills:

Avoid Faulty Thinking — explores how employees view their world and themselves and how these perceptions influence their thinking, feelings and behaviours. Without this insight employees are at risk for continued faulty thinking, such as believing their life can never be any better.

Energy — focuses on stress management strategies and pro-health habits that can influence how one copes with stress. Learning to develop coping skills requires energy. People caught in stress often adopt sedentary lifestyles or unhealthy habits (e.g., smoking, over-eating, etc.) as a way to cope. Proactive action and healthy habits provide energy to cope with life.

Human Behaviour Insights — introduces employees to a user-friendly framework on what motivates most human beings. This gives employees insight on what drives their choices. This module explores how each person is capable of making both effective and less-effective choices. This core competency also introduces the power of emotions in driving behaviour choices.

The second level of this program moves from foundation to developmental skills. These skills focus on teaching employees how to influence their thinking to cope with life's stresses.

Positive Thinking — teaches employees to eliminate limiting beliefs and negative self-talk. This allows them to challenge their thinking and to create new positive thinking that drives new feelings, thoughts and behaviours.

Resilience — introduces resiliency. It provides an exploration of the role of optimism and the benefits of enhancing creativity, problem solving and decision making. Resiliency assists individuals to bounce back from life's potholes so they can dust off and push forward.

Self-confidence — explores the role self-esteem and self-acceptance play in developing self-confidence. A critical element that influences one's ability to cope is belief in oneself. Key building blocks for developing self-esteem are definable and measurable.

The third level of this program deals with mastery skills that influence how effectively employees cope in life.

Relationships — explores the role of relationships in employees' overall ability to cope. Every person who is committed to living a healthy life requires healthy relationships that they can tap into and leverage. Life is more fulfilling when one does not feel they are alone. As a result, there is value in exploring how healthy relationships are and what employees can do to enhance their relationships at work and at home.

Flexibility — explores how flexibility influences employees' ability to adapt and cope with life change and how this can influence their overall well-being. Life is filled with change. To push through life's potholes may require normalizing loss, hopelessness, failure and fear so one can suspend personal judgment and move forward.

Leadership from Within — explores how employees can benefit from evolving their leadership from within to better cope with and manage their life. Actively focusing on self-leadership skills can influence and shape an individual's self-discipline and internal drive to achieve what they define as important. Individuals will be exposed to leadership core competencies that can benefit an employee regardless of their title.

Individuals' coping skills define the degree to which they are able to achieve good outcomes under pressure. This program introduces the pathway to coping but its success depends on employees' motivation and willingness to practice the skills taught. This program has never failed; however, some learners fail to practice and gain the full benefits of the information presented. All concepts taught in this program have been proven and tested over the years and have helped many individuals. In the end, success depends on participants' willingness to be patient and understand that these skills take effort and practice. There are no shortcuts and no silver bullet — only a willingness to learn and grow to achieve full potential.

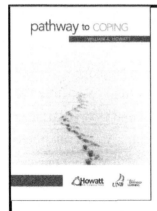

Pathway to Coping

This resource is designed to support the curriculum for a program called *Pathway to Coping* that is designed to help individuals develop their coping skills. The goal is for every learner to develop their coping skills and to become confident that they can achieve life goals such as health, happiness, and productivity.

Nine core competencies for developing coping skills are presented in this book, beginning with a foundational stage of three grounding core competencies.

The second level moves from foundation to developmental skills. These skills focus on teaching employees how to influence their thinking to cope with life's stresses.

The third level deals with mastery skills that influence how effectively employees cope in life.

APPENDIX B

THE GLOBE AND MAIL*

Report on Business: YOUR LIFE AT WORK

http://www.theglobeandmail.com/report-on-business/careers/career-advice/life-at-work/

- **Article 1 in Series — Survey and Quality of Work Life Score (QWL): How's your life at work?**
  http://www.theglobeandmail.com/report-on-business/careers/career-advice/life-at-work/survey-hows-your-life-at-work/article16524403/

- **Article 2 in Series — Your Life at Work Survey: What can a manager do to help an unhappy employee?**
  http://www.theglobeandmail.com/report-on-business/careers/career-advice/life-at-work/what-can-a-manager-do-to-help-an-unhappy-employee/article17070452/

- **Article 3 in Series — Your Life at Work Survey: Is coping with work stress good enough?**
  http://www.theglobeandmail.com/report-on-business/careers/career-advice/life-at-work/is-coping-with-work-stress-good-enough/article17435268/

- **Article 4 in Series — Your Life at Work Survey: When you're unhappy, what motivates you to make a change?**
  http://www.theglobeandmail.com/report-on-business/careers/career-advice/life-at-work/when-youre-unhappy-what-motivates-you-to-make-a-change/article18370595/

- **Article 5 in Series — Your Life at Work Survey: Are you strug-gling to cope with the stress of work and life?**
  http://www.theglobeandmail.com/report-on-business/careers/career-advice/life-at-work/are-you-struggling-to-cope-with-the-stress-of-work-and-life/article18469369/

- **Article 6 in Series — Your Life at Work Survey:: Survey says: We're stressed (and not loving it).**
  http://www.theglobeandmail.com/report-on-business/careers/career-advice/life-at-work/survey-says-were-stressed-and-not-loving-it/article22722102/

- **Article 7 in Series — A lot of Canada's workers are stressed out. But what can be done to fix this?**
  http://www.theglobeandmail.com/report-on-business/video/video-a-lot-of-canadas-workers-are-stressed-out-but-what-can-be-done-to-fix-this/article22738814/

Quality of Life Survey (QL). Are you satisfied with your life?
http://www.theglobeandmail.com/report-on-business/careers/career-advice/life-at-work/are-you-satisfied-with-your-life/article23426459/

Quality of Student Life Survey (QSL). Students: how stressed are you?
http://www.theglobeandmail.com/report-on-business/careers/career-advice/life-at-work/students-how-stressed-are-you/article24378778/

APPENDIX C

Food Addiction Quick Survey

Food addiction can be defined as a compulsion to use food to create mood change (Coombs[29]). Persons with a food addiction use food to feel better, similar to persons addicted to drugs who take drugs with the goal to feel better. It is common for a person with a food addiction to experience withdrawal symptoms such as anxiety, agitation and other negative emotions. Like any addiction, there are risks associated with chronic food addictive behaviour. Persons with food addictions will continue to eat regardless of the negative consequences such as weight gain and damaging personal relationships. The purpose of this survey is to help you self-evaluate your current risk level for food addiction[30].

This is not a clinical measure or diagnostic tool;
it is meant only to be a screening tool.

Over the past six months, how often have you done the following?	Never 0	1 Time	2-3 Times 2	4-5 Times 3	6 or More Times 4
1. Struggled to control how much you ate.					
2. Ate more on days you found stressful.					
3. Ate even when you did not feel hungry.					
4. Noticed food was a source of pleasure.					
5. Lied about your eating.					
6. Craved bread and/or foods high in sugar and salt.					
7. Made excuses to overcome guilt and to rationalize eating.					
8. Planned to eat healthier and failed to follow through.					
9. Sneaked food and ate privately so no one could see you eating.					
10. Felt guilty after you ate.					

Potential Risk Levels		
0-3	**Low Risk**	May not be a concern; however, it is important to monitor your spontaneous eating. Be aware of the relationship between your current stress and eating habits. If you engage in mindless eating when stressed this may be a symptom of ineffective coping skills.
4-10	**Moderate Risk**	At this level you could be at risk for developing a food addiction if you are unaware that you may be beginning to use food to feel better. Ask yourself, "Do I eat to feel better emotionally? Do I have control of my eating?" Digesting excess calories over time will increase body fat. That can result in health conditions such as hypertension, high blood pressure, and obesity. If you eat for emotional comfort this may be a symptom that you are on the road to developing a food addiction or compensating for some other potential mental health issue (e.g., depression). We recommend that if you feel trapped and not sure what to do to call your employee assistance professional, doctor or mental health professional.
11-40	**High Risk**	At this level you are at risk of food controlling your life and you may already have developed a food addiction. We encourage you to self-evaluate and examine your risk for food addiction. There are free, professional, on-line resources that you can access. If you are motivated to get help, there are trained mental health professionals who have expertise in addictions and are ready and willing to help get you on the right path. Like any addiction, the first steps require self-awareness and motivation to take action. A professional or peer support group can help you discover how to take control of food.

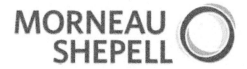

MORNEAU SHEPELL

In 2014, Morneau Shepell began working to integrate its widely used employee health risk assessment survey (HRA); its leading benefit plan consulting approaches and predictive analytics tools with Howatt HR's Quality of Work Life survey designed by Dr. Bill Howatt, Ph.D., Ed.D. Bill's research findings on coping skills show they are a leading indicator for predicting the health and engagement of a workforce and ultimately workforce productivity. In July of 2015, Bill Howatt joined Morneau Shepell as Chief Research and Development Officer for Workforce Productivity.

The combined survey and services represent Morneau Shepell's industry leading analysis and insights to give employers the *what and why* in workplace health. Organizations can build the shared responsibility — between employer and employee — for employee health, engagement and productivity through awareness, accountability and action planning.

About Morneau Shepell Inc.

Morneau Shepell is the only human resources consulting and technology company that takes an integrative approach to employee assistance, health, benefits and retirement needs. The Company is the leading provider of employee and family assistance programs, the largest administrator of retirement and benefits plans and the largest provider of integrated absence management solutions in Canada. Through health and productivity, administrative and retirement solutions, Morneau Shepell helps clients reduce costs, increase employee productivity and improve their competitive position. Established in 1966, Morneau Shepell serves approximately 20,000 clients, ranging from small businesses to some of the largest corporations and associations in North America. With almost 4,000 employees, Morneau Shepell provides services to organizations across Canada, the United States and around the globe. Morneau Shepell is a publicly traded company on the Toronto Stock Exchange (TSX: MSI). For more information, visit morneaushepell.com.

NOTES

Meet the Author

William A. Howatt
Chief Research & Development Officer, Workforce Productivity, Morneau Shepell

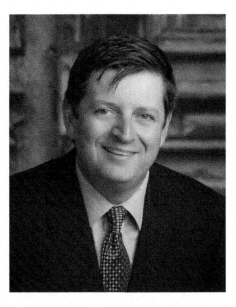

Dr. Bill Howatt has over 25 years' experience in strategic HR, mental health and addictions, and leadership. He has published numerous books and articles, such as *The Coping Crisis, Pathways to Coping, TalOp®: Taking the Guesswork Out of Management,* the *Howatt HR Elements Series,* the *Wiley Series on Addictions, Human Services Counsellor's Toolbox, The Addiction Counsellor's Desk Reference* and *The Addiction Counsellor's Toolbox.* He is the author of *Beyond Engagement: The Employee Care Advantage* and the creator of the Quality of Work Life (QWL) methodology and survey. He is the co-author of behavioural engineering, a strategy aligned to the QWL to provide guidance on how to lead employees to facilitate behavioural change.

He is a regular contributor to *The Globe and Mail* and is behind the Your Life at Work initiative, where there is a miniversion of the QWL that has been explored by more than 10,000 Canadians.

Bill Howatt, Ph.D., Ed.D., Post Doctorate Behavioral Science, University of California, Los Angeles, Semel Institute for Neuro-science and Human Behavior, RTC, RSW, ICADC

CPSIA information can be obtained
at www.ICGtesting.com
Printed in the USA
LVOW04s0530160217
524466LV00001B/1/P